MCQ Tutor for Principles and Practice of Surgery

For Churchill Livingstone

Publisher: Laurence Hunter
Project Editor: Barbara Simmons
Production Controller: Debra Barrie
Design direction: Erik Bigland

MCQ Tutor for Principles and Practice of Surgery

T. Diamond BSc MD FRCSI FRCS
Senior Lecturer
Department of Surgery
Queen's University of Belfast;
Consultant Surgeon
Mater Hospital, Belfast

W.D.B. Clements BSc FRCS
Senior Registrar
Department of Surgery
Queen's University of Belfast

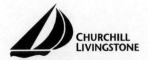

CHURCHILL
LIVINGSTONE

NEW YORK EDINBURGH LONDON MADRID MELBOURNE SAN FRANCISCO
AND TOKYO 1995

CHURCHILL LIVINGSTONE

Medical Division of Pearson Professional Limited

Distributed in the United States of America by Churchill
Livingstone Inc., 650 Avenue of the Americas, New York,
N.Y. 10011, and by associated companies, branches and
representatives throughout the world.

First published 1995

ISBN 0 443 051925

British Library Cataloguing in Publication Data
A catalogue record for this book is available from the British
Library.

Library of Congress Cataloging in Publication Data
A catalog record for this book is available from the Library of
Congress.

The
publisher's
policy is to use
**paper manufactured
from sustainable forests**

Produced by Longman Singapore Publishers Pte Ltd
Printed in Singapore

How to use this book

Multiple choice questions are used ubiquitously at all levels of examination for the undergraduate and postgraduate student and, together with full, explanatory answers, serve as a powerful and efficient revision tool. They test a broad-based knowledge and should stimulate students to explore areas where their knowledge is deficient.

In this MCQ tutor, the sections have been written to accompany the text of *Principles and Practice of Surgery* (Churchill Livingstone, 1995), edited by A.P.M. Forrest, D.C. Carter and I.B. Macleod. Each answer page includes a reference to the appropriate chapter in the textbook. Full explanatory answers are given for the questions, however, so that this book may be used usefully with any surgery book. Information additional to that given in *Principles and Practice of Surgery* is included so that this book is didactic for undergraduate students preparing for final MB and is a useful revision exercise for postgraduate students preparing for the second part of Surgical Fellowship.

The book has been designed with the questions on the right-hand page and the answers on the following left-hand page. We recommend that you answer each section of the book after having revised the relevant section from a main text. Committing yourself to a written answer is an important part of the exercise and time taken to mark the answer is equally important. Each section contains 10 questions with five stems. Give yourself 1 mark for a correct answer, 0 for each you don't know and −1 for each incorrect answer. This permits an accurate assessment of performance and should highlight areas where knowledge is deficient. It should also be informative through the accompanying explanatory statements, and consolidate and reinforce your present knowledge.

We hope this book serves the purpose for which it has been written, and is enjoyed by students of surgery at all levels.

Belfast   T.D.
1995   W.D.B.C.

Acknowledgements

We would like to express our sincere thanks to Mrs Glynis Johnston, Department of Surgery, Queen's University, Belfast, for secretarial assistance, and Laurence Hunter and Barbara Simmons of Churchill Livingstone for their invaluable support.

Abbreviations

ACTH	Adrenocorticotrophic hormone
ADH	Antiduretic hormone
AIDS	Acquired immune deficiency syndrome
APC	Adenomatour polyposis coli
ARDS	Adult respiratory distress syndrome
BCC	Basal cell carcinoma
BMI	Body mass index
BRCA1	Breast cancer gene 1
CBD	Common bile duct
CDAI	Crohn's disease activity index
CEA	Carcino embryonic antigen
CSF	Cerebrospinal fluid
CT	Computerised tomographic (scan)
CVP	Central venous pressure
DIC	Disseminated intravascular coagulation
DMSA	Dimercaptosuccinic acid
DNA	Deoxyribonucleic acid
DO$_2$	Alveolar arterial oxygen tension difference
DPL	Diagnostic peritoneal lavage
DVT	Deep vein thrombosis
ECG	Electrocardiograph
ENT	Ear, nose and throat
ERCP	Endoscopic retrograde cholangio-pancreatography
FAP	Familial adenomatous polyposis
FEV$_1$	Forced expiratory volume in one second
F$_1$O$_2$	Inspired oxygen concentration
FNA	Fine needle aspiration
FVC	Forced vital capacity
HPV	Human papilloma virus
IgE	Immunoglobulin E
INR	International ratio
IVC	Inferior vena cava
IVU	Intravenous urogram
LDH	Lactic dehydrogenase
LHRH	Luteinising hormone releasing hormone
MAC	Minimum alveolar concentration

MEN	Multiple endocrine neoplasia
MIBG	Metaiodobenzoguanidine
MODS	Multiple organ dysfunction syndrome
MRI	Magnetic resonance imaging
NSAID	Non-steroidal anti-inflammatory drug
OGD	Oesophago-gastro-duodenoscopy
OPSI	Overwhelming post-splenectomy infection
PaO₂	Partial pressure of oxygen
PaCO₂	Partial pressure of carbon dioxide
PEEP	Positive end expiratory pressure
PMN	Polymorphonuclear
PTC	Percutaneous transhepatic cholangiogram
PTFE	Polytetrafluroethylene
RNA	Ribo-nucleic acid
SIRS	Systemic inflammatory response syndorme
TPN	Total parenteral nutrition
TURP	Transurethral resection of prostate
UTI	Urinary tract infection
VIP	Vasoactive intestinal peptide
VMA	Vinyl mandelic acid
VO₂	Mixed venous oxygen concentration

Contents

1. The metabolic response to injury

Principles of fluid and electrolyte balance

1 Concerning fluid and electrolyte imbalance:
  - **A** in intestinal obstruction, more fluid is generally lost with higher than with lower obstruction.
  - **B** thirst occurs following a reduction of total body water by 1–2% (350–700 ml).
  - **C** sodium depletion is generally treated by intravenous infusion of hypertonic saline.
  - **D** administration of diuretics may lead to retention of potassium.
  - **E** potassium depletion may result in ECG changes including a decreased QT interval, depressed ST segment and T wave inversion.

2 Concerning normal water and electrolyte balance in an average 70 kg adult:
  - **A** approximately 2000–2500 ml of urine is passed in 24 hours.
  - **B** the major extracellular cation is potassium.
  - **C** approximately 300 ml of fluid is lost in faeces in 24 hours.
  - **D** approximately 1200–1500 ml of fluid is lost as water vapour via the skin and respiratory tract (insensible water loss).
  - **E** aldosterone acts on the kidney to conserve potassium and hydrogen ions.

3 Intravenous administration of normal daily fluid and electrolyte requirements includes:
  - **A** provision of sodium as a 1.8% sodium chloride solution.
  - **B** provision of a total volume of 3.0 litres.
  - **C** administration of an intravenous bolus of 40 mmol of potassium chloride.
  - **D** administration of the average daily sodium requirement as 1 litre of 0.9% sodium chloride.
  - **E** administration of 1 litre of 5% dextrose and 2 litres of 0.9% sodium chloride.

(Answers overleaf)

1 A True   Because fluid secreted by the upper intestinal tract fails to reach the absorptive areas of the distal jejunum, ileum and colon.

B True

C False   Sodium depletion is corrected slowly by intravenous infusion of 0.9% saline. The use of hypertonic saline is only rarely indicated — if the serum sodium has fallen below 110 mmol/l or convulsions have developed.

D False   Diuretic administration may lead to potassium depletion.

E False   Potassium depletion may result in an increased QT interval, ST segment depression and T wave inversion.

2 A False   The figure is 1000–1500 ml in 24 hours.

B False   The major extracellular cation is sodium. Potassium is the major intracellular cation.

C True

D False   The figure is 700–1000 ml.

E False   The action of aldosterone on the kidney involves retention of sodium ions and excretion of potassium and hydrogen ions.

3 A False   Sodium is provided as a 0.9% sodium chloride solution known as normal or physiological saline.

B True   This is the average daily requirement.

C False   Potassium should never be given as an intravenous bolus as cardiac arrest will occur. It is administered as potassium chloride (e.g. 40 mmol added to 1 litre of 5% dextrose or 0.9% saline and given intravenously over 6–8 hours).

D True   This contains 154 mmol of sodium.

E False   Only 1 litre of 0.9% saline is required. The remaining volume (2 litres) should be supplied by 5% dextrose which is an isotonic, non-electrolyte solution.

(For more information, see chs 1 and 2 of Principles and Practice of Surgery)

4 The metabolic response to injury is characterised by a sequence of physiological events aimed at:

A   reducing core body temperature.
B   conservation of sodium and water.
C   mobilising glucose from fat and protein stores.
D   maintaining body weight.
E   enhancing immune function.

5 Precipitating physiological events in the metabolic response to injury include:

A   haemorrhage.
B   pain.
C   ischaemia.
D   endotoxaemia.
E   intestinal obstruction.

6 The catabolic phase of the metabolic response to injury:

A   is independent of the injurious insult.
B   is characterised by an increase in ADH secretion.
C   is characterised by parasympathomimetic overdrive.
D   is impaired in malnourished patients.
E   is potentiated in multiply traumatised patients.

7 The following physiological events occur following injury:

A   urinary output decreases.
B   plasma osmolality decreases.
C   basal metabolic rate increases.
D   urinary excretion of sodium and potassium falls.
E   the patient's blood becomes hypercoagulable.

8 Immediately following a major thermal injury there is a rise in the systemic concentrations of the following substances:

A   insulin.
B   glucagon.
C   growth hormone.
D   testosterone.
E   ACTH.

(Answers overleaf)

4 A False   Body temperature is increased to reduce energy expenditure.
   B True   Volume depletion is frequently the initial injurious insult.
   C True   Gluconeogenesis provides a pool of available glucose for catabolism and ultimately repair.
   D False   Body weight is inevitably reduced during the catabolic phase.
   E True

5 A True   Volume depletion, either externally as in bleeding or following burns, or occult fluid sequestration is frequently the initial insult.
   B True   Afferent impulses on reaching the hypothalamus provoke hormone release and sympathetic outflow.
   C True   Compounded by reperfusion, this initiates the inflammatory response.
   D True   Endotoxaemia is a potent stimulus for the inflammatory cascade.
   E True   By way of volume depletion and endotoxaemia.

6 A False   The greater the magnitude of the injury the greater the catabolic process.
   B True   This aims to restore circulatory volume.
   C False   Increased sympathetic activity.
   D True   These patients have less reserve and therefore have an attenuated response.
   E True

7 A True   Due to ADH secretion.
   B False   Due to Na^+ retention.
   C True   Typical of the catabolic process.
   D False   Potassium excretion is increased.
   E True   Noradrenaline and ADH may increase platelet number and their adhesiveness.

8 A False   Insulin is an anabolic hormone.
   B True   Important initially in providing glucose for energy.
   C True   Present in both the catabolic and anabolic phase in increased concentrations.
   D False   Anabolic hormone secreted in the anabolic phase.
   E True   Important early hormone in the stress response.

(For more information, see chs 1 and 2 of Principles and Practice of Surgery)

9   The average 70 kg adult:

   A has a 24-hour urinary output of 400 ml.

   B ingests 20 g of protein per day.

   C has a basal metabolic rate of 1800 kcal/day.

   D has a 48-hour store of liver glycogen.

   E utilises fat as the main energy source.

10   Patients fasted for more than 24 hours:

   A utilise glucose by glycogenolysis.

   B utilise glucose by gluconeogenesis.

   C utilise ketones as the main cerebral energy source.

   D have an increased basal metabolic rate.

   E will develop hypotension.

(Answers overleaf)

9 A False   About 1000–1500 ml is average. <400 ml = oliguria.
                   <200 ml = anuria.
   B False   This is too low. Average is between 50–100 g.
   C True
   D False   Glycogen stores last only 12–18 hours, and provide
                   the main initial energy source in acute starvation and
                   post injury.
   E False   Fat stores are not usually mobilised unless under
                   stressful circumstances. Carbohydrate usually
                   provides the energy.

10 A True
   B True
   C False   Not until glucose sources are severely depleted
                   (i.e. after 2–3 weeks).
   D False   The BMR remains around 1800 kcal/day and will fall
                   to 1500 kcal after prolonged starvation.
   E False   Blood pressure is maintained until the terminal
                   phases of starvation.

(For more information, see chs 1 and 2 of Principles and Practice of Surgery)

2. Shock

Transfusion of blood and blood products

11 Causes of hypovolaemic shock include:
- **A** burn injury.
- **B** intestinal fistulae.
- **C** spinal cord transection.
- **D** myocardial infarction.
- **E** endotoxaemia.

12 Clinical features of shock include:
- **A** a low cardiac output in the majority of cases.
- **B** a rapid thready pulse.
- **C** a decreased respiratory rate.
- **D** a fall in urine output.
- **E** warm clammy extremities in the majority of cases.

13 Management of hypovolaemic shock involves:
- **A** achievement of venous access via peripheral vein catheterisation.
- **B** bladder catheterisation.
- **C** immediate administration of whole blood or red cell concentrate.
- **D** avoidance of narcotic analgesic agents.
- **E** oxygen administration.

(Answers overleaf)

11 A True   Due to direct fluid loss from the burn and tissue fluid sequestration.

  B True   Due to gastrointestinal fluid loss. This may also occur with severe vomiting or diarrhoea and following sequestration of fluid in the bowel lumen in intestinal obstruction.

  C False   This leads to neurogenic shock due to loss of sympathetic outflow and subsequent vasodilatation.

  D False   This may lead to cardiogenic shock due to 'pump failure'.

  E False   This leads to 'endotoxic' or 'septic' shock, in which the principal event is a fall in systemic vascular resistance due to loss of vascular tone, which occurs secondary to release of various inflammatory mediators (e.g. cytokines).

12 A True   The exception is septic shock, where the cardiac output is usually high secondary to a fall in systemic vascular resistance.

  B True

  C False   The respiratory rate is increased due to acidosis and chemoreceptor stimulation.

  D True   Due to decreased renal perfusion.

  E False   The extremities are usually cold except in septic shock where they may be warm due to peripheral vasodilatation.

13 A True   Two wide-bore peripheral cannulae (e.g. antecubital fossae) should be used initially. Later, a central venous catheter should be inserted to allow measurement of the CVP.

  B True   The urinary catheter should be connected to an hourly 'urometer' to allow accurate measurement of urinary output.

  C False   'Colloid' or 'crystalloid' solutions may be used initially. Blood or red cell concentrate may be given later, after cross-matching, but in extreme situations, uncrossed group O rhesus-negative blood may be used.

  D False   Effective analgesia should not be withheld from hypovolaemic patients.

  E True

(For more information, see chs 3 and 4 of Principles and Practice of Surgery)

14 Complications of blood transfusion include:
  A   an acute haemolytic transfusion reaction.
  B   a febrile reaction.
  C   cardiac failure.
  D   hypercalcaemia.
  E   thrombocytosis.

15 Stored whole blood used for transfusion:
  A   contains similar amounts of coagulation factors as normal blood.
  B   contains a concentration of leucocytes similar to that of normal blood.
  C   can be stored for up to 100 days at 4±2°C.
  D   is sterile.
  E   is used when rapid volume transfusion is required in a patient who has suffered major trauma.

16 Shock:
  A   is defined as an acute decrease in circulating blood volume.
  B   may occur in the presence of normotension.
  C   may occur following cardiomyopathy.
  D   may follow gastrointestinal perforation.
  E   invariably results in sympathomimetic activity in the arteriolar circulation.

(Answers overleaf)

14 A True   This is usually due to ABO incompatibility and usually caused by errors in identification of the patient.

  B True   This is common, particularly in patients who have had multiple transfusions. It should be treated by stopping the infusion and administering an antipyretic agent (e.g. paracetamol 500–1000 mg).

  C True   Particularly in chronically anaemic or elderly patients. The problem may be reduced by giving i.v. frusemide (40 mg) with alternate units of blood.

  D False   Hypocalcaemia may occur, particularly with large volume transfusion, due to the citrate used in blood as an anticoagulant. This can bind ionised calcium.

  E False   Thrombocytopenia may occur with large volume transfusion as stored blood does not contain functional platelets.

15 A False   Stored blood contains very little factor V and VIII but has other factors in adequate amounts for haemostasis. Red cell concentrate provides only small amounts of coagulation factors.

  B False   Stored blood contains very few leucocytes.

  C False   It may be stored for up to 30 days at $4\pm2°C$.

  D False   Blood is not sterilised and can therefore transmit organisms if these have not been detected by donor screening.

  E True

16 A False   Shock occurs when cellular perfusion is inadequate resulting in decreased delivery of oxygen and other vital substrates with decreased removal of waste products. In some cases of shock, the circulating blood volume may be normal.

  B True

  C True   Cardiogenic shock.

  D True   Gastrointestinal perforation may result in major fluid and electrolyte disturbances and ultimately sepsis.

  E False   In septic shock, vasodilatation is characteristic.

(For more information, see chs 3 and 4 of Principles and Practice of Surgery)

17 Septic shock:

  A occurs most commonly following systemic infection with Gram-negative aerobic organisms.
  B usually has its offending organism retrieved by standard bacteriological methods.
  C may occur secondary to hypovolaemic shock.
  D results in decreased activation of mononuclear cells of the immune system.
  E may result in arteriovenous shunting within the microcirculation.

18 Anaphylactic shock:

  A is an immune-mediated reaction.
  B results in mast cell activation and increased circulating histamine concentrations.
  C produces microcirculatory changes similar to hypovolaemic shock.
  D requires prompt treatment with parenteral adrenaline and hydrocortisone.
  E may occur after ingestion of drugs.

19 In circulatory shock:

  A myocardial contractility is enhanced.
  B the ensuing metabolic acidosis is well compensated by the kidneys' ability to excrete H^+ ions and preserve HCO_3^-.
  C red cell deformability is increased, while margination of neutrophils is decreased.
  D the patient's coagulation time may be adversely effected, especially if due to a septic insult.
  E failure to correct the process may result in resistant pulmonary oedema with reduced pulmonary compliance.

(Answers overleaf)

17 A True   Usually Gram-negative bacilli; however,
Gram-positive organisms and fungi may also be
implicated.

B False   An organism is rarely recovered. The diagnosis of
the systemic inflammatory response syndrome
(SIRS) is based on other parameters.

C True   Hypoperfusion of the intestinal tract will result in a
breach in mucosal integrity and bacterial
translocation.

D False   Mononuclear cells are activated and secrete
proinflammatory cytokines.

E True   This is a characteristic physiological occurrence in
sepsis, with resultant microcirculatory disturbance
and local tissue hypoxia.

18 A True   Type I hypersensitivity (IgE-mediated reaction).

B True   Mast cells are ubiquitously located at the body's
internal/external interface, where they are
strategically situated to interact with foreign
allergens.

C False   More similar to those seen in septic shock, i.e. a
massive fall in systemic venous resistance with
increased capillary permeability.

D True   It is a medical emergency requiring expeditious
administration of adrenaline, steroids and
antihistamines.

E True   For example, penicillin, also iodine-based
radiological contrast medium.

19 A False   Sympathetic drive may increase the heart rate, but
local metabolic acidosis will adversely affect the
performance of the myocardium.

B False   Renal hypoperfusion alters the ability of the kidney
to compensate.

C False   Red cells have a decreased ability to deform and
neutrophil margination increases; both changes
contribute to plugging of small capillaries and
consequently local hypoxia.

D True   Although coagulation is enhanced in most forms of
shock due to increased viscosity and stimulation of
the coagulation cascade. Microcirculatory platelet
plugging and disseminated intravascular coagulation
results in a consumption coagulopathy.

E True   These are features of ARDS.

(For more information, see chs 3 and 4 of Principles and Practice of Surgery)

20 In uncontrolled sepsis requiring intensive supportive management:

A long-term antibiotic therapy is an essential treatment strategy.

B pulmonary artery flotation catheters are inserted to define the oxygen extraction ratio.

C increasing blood lactate level is correlated with mortality.

D inotropic support is detrimental to the already compromised splanchnic circulation.

E adult respiratory distress syndrome is best treated by mechanical ventilation with positive end expiratory pressure (PEEP).

(Answers overleaf)

20 **A** **False**   This may result in systemic candidiasis which has considerable mortality.
    B **True**   This can be calculated from the VO_2 and DO_2.
    C **True**   This reflects the degree of metabolic acidosis.
    D **False**   Inotropes are ubiquitously used in promoting renal blood flow and increasing blood pressure.
    E **True**

(For more information, see chs 3 and 4 of Principles and Practice of Surgery)

3. Nutritional support in surgical patients

Investigation and diagnosis of surgical patients

21 Preoperative nutritional status can be assessed from:

  A body weight.
  B serum transferrin concentration.
  C blood sugar concentration.
  D tricipital skin fold thickness.
  E differential leucocyte count.

22 Basic nutritional requirements in a 70 kg adult:

  A include 140 g of carbohydrate per day.
  B include 14 g of nitrogen per day.
  C decrease in the presence of Crohn's disease with a high enterocutaneous fistula.
  D who is starving are decreased as regards total energy requirements.
  E decrease if the patient is mechanically ventilated.

23 Enteral feeding:

  A is contraindicated in patients with pseudobulbar palsy.
  B is contraindicated in mechanically ventilated patients.
  C has advantages over parenteral feeding in the multiply traumatised patient.
  D promotes bacterial translocation from the gastrointestinal tract.
  E may be complicated by lobar pneumonia.

(Answers overleaf)

21 A True   Body mass index $\left(\dfrac{body\ weight}{height^2}\right)$ gives an accurate reflection of nutritional status. BMI <20 suggests malnourishment, and <15 means the patient is dangerously malnourished.

  B True   Depressed visceral protein concentration infers severe malnourishment.

  C False   Blood sugar levels are maintained in malnourishment.

  D False   This measurement only reflects body fat content. Mid-arm muscle circumference, however, gives an accurate reflection of lean body mass.

  E True   Lymphopenia <1.2 × 10^9/l is a useful marker of impaired nutritional status.

22 A True

  B False   The normal daily requirement for nitrogen is 7 g/24 h. However, patients who are catabolic following injury may require up to 30 g of nitrogen per day.

  C False   Loss of enteric content implies loss of calories which necessitates dietary supplementation.

  D True   Although energy requirement is less, the proportion of nitrogen required daily is increased.

  E False   More energy is required to recover the increased insensible heat and water loss.

23 A False   Percutaneous endoscopic gastrostomy tubes are frequently employed in patients with an absent gag reflex.

  B False   Fine-bore nasogastric or jejunostomy tube feeding is a popular method of feeding in unconscious patients.

  C True   Enteral feeding prevents intestinal mucosal atrophy. NB: When the gut is available, use it!

  D False   Enteral feeding helps preserve the intestinal mucosa and barrier function.

  E True   Aspiration pneumonitis is the major complication in nasogastric enteral feeding.

(For more information, see chs 5 and 6 of Principles and Practice of Surgery)

24 Parenteral nutrition:
    A cannot be administered via the cephalic vein.
    B can provide the patient's entire requirement of protein,
       energy, electrolytes, trace metals and vitamins.
    C in the form of 20% lipid emulsion is an inefficient energy
       source in the septic patient.
    D via the subclavian vein can cause axillary vein thrombosis.
    E can result in cholestatic hyperbilirubinaemia.

25 Concerning the use of a central venous catheter:
    A administration of TPN is safe and does not require repetitive
       haematological and biochemical monitoring.
    B its insertion should have mandatory electrocardiographic
       monitoring.
    C it provides a convenient portal for blood sampling and
       antibiotic administration.
    D if tunnelled subcutaneously it has a higher incidence of
       infection with endogenous staphylococcus.
    E if infected it is effectively treated by administration of
       antibiotics via the offending catheter.

**26 Preoperative histological and cytological investigations
include:**
    A fine-needle aspiration of lumps (e.g. breast, thyroid) for
       histological examination.
    B Tru-cut needle biopsy for histological examination.
    C Crosby capsule biopsy of the colonic mucosa.
    D punch biopsy of gastric or colonic mucosa.
    E exfoliative cytology to detect cells from lung tumours.

(Answers overleaf)

24 A False   Lipid emulsion and isotonic solutions of amino acids are available which can be administered via a peripheral vein. Vein half-life can be prolonged with the use of topical nitroglycerine patches.

B True   Hence the term total parenteral nutrition (TPN).

C False   Septic patients have difficulty metabolising glucose, hence fat is an excellent energy substrate.

D True   Thrombophlebitis due to infusion of hypertonic solutions is a well-recognised complication.

E True   Long-term administration of lipid emulsions can cause cholestatic liver dysfunction with jaundice.

25 A False   Many biochemical disturbances may occur, therefore regular measurements of blood urea, electrolytes, full blood picture, liver function tests, blood glucose, serum albumin, calcium, magnesium and phosphate are mandatory.

B True   Life-threatening ventricular arrhythmias may occur following injudicious central venous catheter placement.

C False   The central line is 'sacrosanct' and should be used exclusively for feeding if sepsis rates are to be kept to a minimum.

D False   This is one method of reducing endogenous line sepsis.

E False   This is ineffective and can be positively dangerous by promoting bacterial resistance and overgrowth of infective agents, e.g. *Candida albicans*.

26 A False   Fine-needle aspiration only obtains cells suitable for cytological assessment. (Cytology refers to examination of the architecture of cells.)

B True   A Tru-cut needle obtains a core of tissue upon which histological examination can be performed. (Histology refers to examination of tissue and its cellular components.)

C False   A Crosby capsule is used to obtain samples of small bowel mucosa.

D True   Punch biopsy is used to obtain tissue from the skin or within the mouth and tissues accessible to endoscopy (e.g. gastroscopy, sigmoidoscopy, colonoscopy).

E True   Exfoliative cytology involves examination of cells shed by epithelium. Cells can be obtained from secretions or excretions (e.g. sputum or urine).

(For more information, see chs 5 and 6 of Principles and Practice of Surgery)

27 Preoperative investigation and preparation of a patient with obstructive jaundice should include:

A measurement of coagulation status.
B measurement of 24-hour urinary output.
C measurement of serum urea and electrolytes.
D fluid restriction during the 24 hours preoperatively.
E administration of antibiotics during invasive diagnostic procedures (e.g. PTC, ERCP)

28 Contrast radiological investigative techniques include:

A a barium meal to investigate the stomach and small bowel.
B a small bowel enema to investigate the colon and rectum.
C a barium swallow to investigate dysphagia.
D a single contrast barium enema to detect small colonic polyps.
E an intravenous cholangiogram to investigate obstructive jaundice.

(Answers overleaf)

27 A True Plus administration of vitamin K if the prothrombin time is prolonged.

B True Some patients with obstructive jaundice may have impaired renal function preoperatively (hepatorenal syndrome).

C True Obstructive jaundice results in hypodypsia. These patients may be dehydrated with an elevated serum urea, and require preoperative i.v. fluid administration to correct this.

D False Approximately 3 litres of fluid should be given intravenously during the 24 hours preoperatively to help ensure adequate hydration and urine flow during the perioperative period.

E True In order to reduce the risk of infection in the obstructed biliary system (cholangitis).

28 A False A barium meal investigates the stomach and proximal duodenum only.

B False A small bowel enema investigates the small intestine. Barium is instilled directly into the small bowel via a tube placed in the duodenum, thus avoiding the need to await gastric emptying.

C True This investigates the oesophagus and may detect motility disorders such as achalasia or obstructive lesions such as carcinoma.

D False A double contrast barium enema is required to detect small colonic polyps. Instillation of both barium and air allows coating of the colonic mucosa with a thin film of barium, hence increasing the chance of detecting polyps.

E False Contrast introduced into the body via the oral route (oral cholecystogram) or intravenous route (i.v. cholangiogram) has to be conjugated with bilirubin and excreted by the liver before it can outline the biliary system. In obstructive jaundice this cannot occur and contrast must be introduced directly into the biliary system as in a percutaneous transhepatic cholangiogram (PTC) or endoscopic retrograde cholangio-pancreatogram (ERCP).

(For more information, see chs 5 and 6 of Principles and Practice of Surgery)

**29 Preoperative investigation and preparation should
    include:**

A an ECG in all patients over 40 years.
B a chest X-ray in all patients over 50 years.
C multichannel biochemical analysis (block analysis) in all
    patients undergoing general anaesthesia.
D a haemoglobin and white cell count in all patients.
E a detailed history and physical examination.

30 In the fasting patient postoperatively:

A the normal intravenous requirement of sodium and chloride
    is 154 mmol/day.
B potassium replacement is required initially.
C if pyrexic is present as much as 5 litres of fluid can be
    required per day.
D intestinal ileus may result from injudicious electrolyte
    replacement.
E with an enterocutaneous fistula, additional fluid in
    the form of 5% dextrose is present is required.

(Answers overleaf)

29 **A** **False**   A routine preoperative ECG is only indicated in elderly patients (>60) or where there is a specific indication (e.g. hypertension, arrhythmias, cardiac failure).

B **False**   A routine preoperative chest X-ray should only be performed in elderly patients (>60) or where there is a specific indication (e.g. history of asthma, chronic cough).

C **False**   This is expensive and only indicated in selected cases (e.g. obstructive jaundice, renal dysfunction).

D **False**   Again, only indicated in specific circumstances. In general, patients undergoing routine surgery tend to be over-investigated; e.g. a healthy 30-year-old male undergoing a hernia operation does not need an ECG, chest X-ray, biochemical analysis, etc.

E **True**   To ensure that the patient is fit for surgery and general anaesthesia and also to detect coincidental disease.

30 **A** **True**

B **False**   Serum potassium concentrations are increased postoperatively and replacement is not usually necessary for at least 48 hours.

C **True**   200 ml/°C/day — sweating and increased respiratory rate all add to the insensible water loss.

D **True**   In prolonged fasting, imbalance in K^+, Ca^{++} and Mg^{++} may produce ileus. There are many other causes.

E **False**   It is important to measure these losses and replace them with normal saline as opposed to isotonic dextrose which is metabolised to water.

(For more information, see chs 5 and 6 of Principles and Practice of Surgery)

4. Infections and antibiotics

31 Factors which predispose to wound infection include:
A impaired blood supply.
B development of a wound haematoma.
C the presence of devitalised tissue in the wound.
D antibiotic administration during surgery.
E foreign material in the wound.

32 Concerning skin and wound infection:
A erysipelas is caused by *Staphylococcus aureus*.
B carbuncles are usually due to staphylococcal infection.
C cellulitis is often caused by streptococcal infection.
D progressive bacterial gangrene (Meleney's gangrene) involves the skin, deep fascia and muscles.
E gas gangrene is caused by *Clostridium perfringens*.

33 The classification of surgical wounds in terms of the risk of postoperative infection includes:
A clean wounds, which are those used to operate on one of the body tracts (e.g. gastrointestinal tract).
B potentially contaminated wounds, which are those used to operate on one of the body tracts.
C contaminated wounds, which are those used to operate on one of the body tracts without adequate preoperative preparation.
D dirty wounds, which include some due to farming accidents and those used to drain pus.
E clean wounds, which should be associated with an infection rate of less than 2%.

34 Concerning surgical antisepsis:
A disinfection refers to complete removal or inactivation of viable microorganisms.
B instruments may be rendered sterile by wet heat at 100°C for 20 minutes.
C the skin may be sterilised by a 1–2% iodine solution painted on before surgery.
D the use of face masks by operating surgeons dramatically reduces the incidence of wound infection.
E instruments may be rendered sterile by dry heat in an oven at 160°C for 1 hour.

(Answers overleaf)

31 A True   This may occur when wounds are closed under tension. In contrast, wounds in skin with an excellent blood supply (e.g. scalp) rarely become infected.

   B True

   C True   Such wounds (e.g. following trauma) are best debrided and left open and then sutured 4–5 days later (delayed primary suture).

   D False   In appropriate situations, 'prophylactic' antibiotic administration is indicated and reduces the risk of wound infection.

   E True

32 A False   The causative organism is streptococcus.

   B True

   C True   Streptococcus may produce a hyaluronidase which accentuates spread of the organism.

   D False   It involves the skin only. Necrotising fasciitis (Fournier's gangrene) involves the subcutaneous tissue and deep fascia.

   E True   Previously called *Clostridium welchii*.

33 A False   Clean wounds do not involve surgery to any of the body tracts (e.g. mastectomy, inguinal hernia repair) — prophylactic antibiotics are indicated only if prosthetic material is to be inserted (e.g. mesh hernia repair).

   B True   Examples include colorectal resection (following adequate preoperative clearance of the bowel) and gastrectomy — prophylactic antibiotics are indicated.

   C True   For example, acute colonic resection for colonic obstruction due to tumour — prophylactic antibiotics are indicated.

   D True   These wounds are generally left open (e.g. incision and drainage of an abscess) or may be closed after 3–4 days (delayed primary suture) — prophylactic antibiotics are NOT indicated, as the wound is left open.

   E True

34 A False   This is the definition of sterilisation. Disinfection refers to a significant reduction in the numbers of organisms present, particularly those which might cause infection.

   B False   121°C is necessary.

   C False   It may be disinfected in this way.

   D False   Several large prospective trials have shown that the wearing of face masks has no significant influence on wound infection rates.

   E True

(For more information, see ch 7 of Principles and Practice of Surgery)

35 Concerning infection following surgery:
  A the risk of chest infection is generally lower following laparoscopic surgery.
  B bacterial colonisation of indwelling urinary catheters eventually occurs.
  C chest infection should be treated by bed rest and antibiotics.
  D antibiotics should be given to all patients with an abdominal wound.
  E all patients with a central venous line should receive prophylactic antibiotics.

36 Wound infection:
  A occurs most commonly after exogenous microbial challenge.
  B may result in leucopenia.
  C rate following elective hernia repair is reduced if it is performed as a day procedure.
  D rate is increased in patients who are greater than 30% under or over their expected weight.
  E is less serious when the offending inoculum contains mixed organisms.

37 Antibiotic prophylaxis:
  A is unnecessary in laparoscopic hernia repair.
  B has reduced the incidence of anastomotic leaks and intraperitoneal abscess following colonic resection.
  C is the primary treatment strategy in a pelvic abscess.
  D is emphasised in patients with acute appendicitis.
  E is unnecessary in patients with a xenograft valve undergoing dental treatment.

(Answers overleaf)

35 A True   Due to reduced pain and improved chest and diaphragmatic excursion.

    B True   Virtually all urinary catheters become colonised with coliform or other organisms within 3–4 days — hence urinary catheters should be removed as early as possible.

    C False   Chest infection should be treated by active mobilisation, aggressive physiotherapy and antibiotics.

    D False   Widespread or indiscriminate antibiotic usage is condemned as it increases the risk of development of antibiotic resistance.

    E False   For the same reason as in **D**.

36 A False   The majority of wound infections are endogenously acquired.

    B True   Polymorphonuclear leucocytosis is more common; however, serious infection may result in a lowered white cell count.

    C True   Reducing inpatient hospital stay reduces the risk of hospital acquired (nosocomial) infections.

    D True   Morbid obesity and malnutrition impair host immune function and predispose patients to septic complications.

    E False   Synergistic infections are extremely serious and may result in enhanced aggression and virulence.

37 A False   This procedure employs the insertion of a nonabsorbable prosthetic mesh.

    B False   The aim of antibiotic prophylaxis is to reduce the incidence of wound infection and deep intracavity infection.

    C False   The primary strategy is to drain the abscess, as with any collection of pus.

    D True   This is one of the commonest 'potentially infected' wounds. Metronidazole administered systemically or rectally will reduce the incidence of wound infection.

    E False   Although patients with a porcine valve in situ do not require antithromboembolic prophylaxis, they always require antibiotic prophylaxis when bacteraemic insult is anticipated.

(For more information, see ch 7 of Principles and Practice of Surgery)

38 Tetanus:

   A is a preventable disease.

   B occurs following contamination with an aerobic spore-forming bacillus.

   C presentation is acute and frequently life-threatening within 24 hours.

   D is successfully treated with a long-acting penicillin.

   E in its full-blown form requires the patient to be fully curarised and ventilated.

39 The following are positive steps in reducing wound infection rates after colonic surgery:

   A antibiotic administration with induction of anaesthesia.

   B skin shaving on the night prior to surgery.

   C colonic cleansing with oral administration of a balanced electrolyte solution.

   D an increased preoperative hospital stay.

   E oral neomycin.

40 Antibiotic prophylaxis:

   A is used solely to prevent wound infection.

   B is only effective when administered parenterally.

   C is safe as the antibiotic is only administered for a limited period.

   D is only used in potentially infected wounds.

   E is only useful when given as a combination of agents.

(Answers overleaf)

38 A True   This requires well-developed medical services, excellent wound management and efficient programmes of active immunisation.

  B False   This is an anaerobic organism which thrives in circumstances where there is necrotic tissue and hypoxia.

  C False   The clinical presentation is frequently insidious and the incubation period may be as long as several months following the initial surgery.

  D False   Successful treatment requires wound debridement as the primary strategy, neutralisation of the neurotoxin with at least 10 000 units of human tetanus immune globulin, antibiotics and intensive supportive therapy.

  E True   Tracheostomy is frequently indicated, and full neuromuscular blockade is used to overcome painful muscle spasms.

39 A True   Prophylactic antibiotic therapy has been a major advance in preventing wound infection.

  B False   Skin shaving 24 hours prior to surgery may be positively harmful as the epidermal barrier is frequently breached.

  C True   This is the most popular method of colonic purgation in preparation for surgery.

  D False   This may increase wound infection rates, especially with nosocomial organisms.

  E True   This will reduce the intraluminal bacterial floral count.

40 A False   When given prior to percutaneous transhepatic cholangiography the aim is to prevent cholangitis.

  B False   Metronidazole is frequently administered rectally and has been shown to be as effective as the intravenous route.

  C False   Antibiotics are dangerous. One dose can result in fatal anaphylactic shock.

  D False   It is used in clean operations (e.g. internal fixation of fractures, valve replacement) where infection would be catastrophic.

  E False   Single agents are used in certain circumstances, e.g. metronidazole is effective in appendicitis and a cephalosporin is adequate in biliary surgery. A bactericidal antibiotic should always be used.

(For more information, see ch 7 of Principles and Practice of Surgery)

5. Pre-operative assessment and preparation

Anaesthesia and the operation

41 A detailed drug history is important preoperatively, particularly to prevent the following associated drug side effects and risks during operation:

- **A** digoxin may cause cardiovascular instability and arrhythmias.
- **B** steroid administered preoperatively may be associated with excess steroid production in the per- and postoperative phases.
- **C** hypotension during anaesthetic induction may occur in patients taking beta blockers.
- **D** clonidine may be associated with rebound hypertension following its withdrawal.
- **E** thiazide diuretics may produce hepatic enzyme induction.

42 The American Society of Anesthesiologists' (ASA) system for classifying anaesthetic risk in terms of physical status includes:

- **A** Class I, referring to a normal healthy individual with no physiological or biochemical disturbances.
- **B** Class II, referring to a patient with severe systemic disease which is not incapacitating (e.g. heart disease with limited exercise tolerance).
- **C** Class IV, referring to a patient with severe, incapacitating systemic disease that is a constant potential threat to life.
- **D** Class V, referring to a moribund patient who is not expected to live.
- **E** Class E, added to denote a patient who requires an emergency operation.

(Answers overleaf)

41 A True
    B False Steroid administration preoperatively may produce suppression of the pituitary-adrenal axis resulting in adrenocorticoid insufficiency in the perioperative period. Such patients should receive i.v. steroids during the pre- and postoperative periods.
    C True
    D True
    E False This is true of barbiturate drugs.

42 A True
    B False This is Class III. Class II refers to mild-to-moderate systemic disease (e.g. hypertension).
    C True For example, congestive heart failure, severe and persistent angina.
    D True In this case, surgery is performed as a last resort (e.g. ruptured aortic aneurysm).
    E True

(For more information, see chs 8 and 9 of Principles and Practice of Surgery)

43 Concerning preoperative assessment and preparation of respiratory function:

A a chest X-ray is indicated in all patients undergoing general anaesthesia.

B diagnosis of respiratory failure is made when the arterial oxygen tension (PaO_2) falls below 60 mmHg.

C type 1 respiratory failure occurs when the arterial carbon dioxide tension ($PaCO_2$) is less than 50 mmHg.

D an FEV_1/FVC ratio of less than 70% indicates significant pulmonary dysfunction.

E intensive physiotherapy with postural drainage and bronchodilators is indicated in patients with chronic chest disease.

44 Concerning preoperative assessment and preparation of the cardiovascular system:

A an ECG should be performed in all patients >45 years.

B blood pressure should be carefully monitored.

C antihypertensive drugs should be continued up to the time of surgery.

D patients taking beta blockers are at risk of tachycardia and bronchoconstriction.

E within 6 months following myocardial infarction, the risk of reinfarction during elective surgical procedures is increased by 10%.

45 The following drugs should be discontinued prior to surgery:

A warfarin.

B aspirin.

C adalat.

D corticosteroids.

E thiazide diuretics.

(Answers overleaf)

43 A False   This is only indicated in specific cases (e.g. history of asthma, chronic cough).
** B False**   The level is 50 mmHg.
** C True**   The $PaCO_2$ is used to subdivide respiratory failure into type 1 ($PaCO_2 < 50$ mmHg) and type 2 ($PaCO_2 > 50$ mmHg). Type 2 failure denotes the presence of CO_2 retention which occurs in severe pulmonary dysfunction.
** D True**
** E True**   This helps clear inspissated secretions from the airways.

44 A False   Only when there is a history or signs of myocardial ischaemia and in elderly patients (>60 years).
** B True**   In significantly hypertensive patients (e.g. diastolic pressure > 100 mmHg), elective surgery should be postponed until the blood pressure is controlled.
** C True**
** D False**   Risks include bradycardia, heart block, congestive cardiac failure and bronchoconstriction.
** E False**   It is increased by 30%. Elective surgery should be postponed by at least 6 months.

45 A True   If anticoagulation is essential, heparin may be used. In some situations (e.g. surgery for peripheral vascular disease) warfarin may be continued.
** B True**   Aspirin can result in haematoma formation after surgery.
** C False**   This is an antihypertensive and should be continued until the time of surgery.
** D False**   If steroids are discontinued abruptly, adrenocortical insufficiency may occur.
** E False**   These can be used safely until the time of surgery.

(For more information, see chs 8 and 9 of Principles and Practice of Surgery)

46 In general anaesthesia:
  A the principal aim is to produce reversible loss of awareness.
  B muscle relaxation is essential.
  C the minimum alveolar concentration (MAC) of an inhalational agent is the tension (kPa) which prevents 50% of the population, given the agent, from responding to painful stimuli.
  D nitrous oxide has an excellent synergistic action with the modern halogenated volatile inhalational agents.
  E patients require mechanical ventilation for the operative period.

47 In general anaesthesia:
  A exhaled CO_2 is rebreathed safely and stimulates respiration.
  B there are four recognised stages of consciousness of which stage 3 is the depth of anaesthesia required for surgical intervention.
  C pulse oximetry is routinely employed to record heart rate and oxygen saturation.
  D suxamethonium is a long-acting non-depolarising muscle relaxant used in maintenance anaesthesia.
  E muscle relaxation induced by curare-based drugs is reversed with atropine.

48 In general anaesthesia:
  A prior to induction it is essential that the stomach is empty of contents.
  B preoperative starvation ensures that the stomach is empty.
  C administration of morphine ensures rapid gastric emptying.
  D the main advantage of the laryngeal mask is that it protects the patient from aspiration pneumonitis.
  E if aspiration pneumonitis occurs it should be treated with vigorous bronchial lavage and systemic steroids.

(Answers overleaf)

46 A True   The other aim is to produce analgesia.
   B False   Patients can breathe spontaneously during the
         operation. Muscle relaxation is mainly used in
         abdominal surgery where access to the peritoneal
         cavity is required.
   C True   A gold standard definition in anaesthesia.
   D False   There is no synergism between anaesthetic agents,
         therefore fractions of the MAC can be added together
         when combinations of inhalational agents are used.
   E False   See explanation in **B**.

47 A False   This is positively dangerous. CO_2 should be absorbed
         by soda lime before exhaled gases can be safely
         rebreathed. It is also possible, with modern
         anaesthetic machines, to have exhaled gas
         discharged by an appropriate arrangement of valves.
   B True
   C True   This is ubiquitously used in anaesthesia and where
         patients are sedated. It provides useful information
         but is not a panacea for patient monitoring.
   D False   Suxamethonium is short-acting (5–10 mins). It is
         used initially when patients are being intubated.
   E False   Neostigmine, an anticholinesterase, is used to
         reverse these drugs. Atropine is usually given to
         block the muscarinic effects of acetylcholine, e.g.
         bradycardia, bronchospasm.

48 A False   This is frequently not possible in emergency
         situations where surgery requires to be performed
         expeditiously. Rapid sequence induction is employed
         and cricoid pressure used to reduce the risk of
         aspiration.
   B False   Gastric emptying is very variable and fasting does
         not guarantee an empty stomach.
   C False   Morphine analgesia delays gastric emptying.
   D False   Its attraction lies in the ease of insertion. It does not
         prevent regurgitation and aspiration.
   E False   Therapeutic bronchoscopy is beneficial; however,
         vigorous lavage may only act to disseminate the
         foreign material. Steroids have little place and it is
         widely accepted that they increase the risks of Gram-
         negative infection.

(For more information, see chs 8 and 9 of Principles and Practice of Surgery)

49 Local anaesthesia:
  A blocks transmission of nerve impulses by altering membrane permeability.
  B only affects sensory nerve fibres.
  C requires infiltration into the subcutaneous tissue to take effect.
  D in high doses can cause convulsions and resistant bradycardia.
  E works well for incision and drainage of subcutaneous abscesses.

50 Regional anaesthesia:
  A by controlled administration of a short-acting local anaesthetic agent is an excellent technique permitting simple surgical procedures on the upper and lower limbs.
  B can be obtained by infiltration of the potential space between the ligamentum flavum and the dura mater of the spinal column with local anaesthetic agents.
  C by spinal infiltration can result in profound hypotension and bradycardia.
  D by spinal infiltration reduces blood loss during surgery, and minimises the risk of deep venous thrombosis.
  E is potentiated by the addition of opioid derivatives.

(Answers overleaf)

49 **A** **True**   It depolarises the membrane of the nerve, preventing conduction.

B **False**   It affects mixed nerves; however, the finer sensory fibres are more susceptible in the doses routinely employed.

C **False**   Topical anaesthesia is used frequently, e.g. prior to venepuncture in children, in catheterisation and to anaesthetise the pharynx prior to oesophago-gastroduodenoscopy (OGD).

D **True**   It is very important to be aware of toxicity from local anaesthesia. CNS excitability and cardiotoxicity are the major complications.

E **False**   Local anaesthesia is of limited use in abscesses, where the acid environment inhibits its action.

50 **A** **True**   Bier's block is an excellent method of regional anaesthesia. One must be extremely cautious that local anaesthetic does not leak into the systemic circulation.

B **True**   This is extradural or epidural anaesthesia.

C **True**   Secondary to sympathetic blockade with decreased vasomotor tone.

D **True**   By sympathetic blockade, peripheral blood flow is increased.

E **True**   This is a relatively novel innovation and permits lower doses of local anaesthesia to be used, hence reducing the risk of toxicity.

(For more information, see chs 8 and 9 of Principles and Practice of Surgery)

6. Postoperative care and complications

Special problems in surgical care

51 In patients with obstructive jaundice:
- **A** the prothrombin time is often reduced.
- **B** there is an increased incidence of renal dysfunction.
- **C** endotoxaemia may occur.
- **D** fluid retention in the extracellular fluid compartment often occurs.
- **E** there is an increased incidence of infective complications.

52 Increased bleeding during surgery may be due to:
- **A** aspirin therapy.
- **B** excessive administration of protamine sulphate.
- **C** thrombocytopenia.
- **D** fibrinolysis.
- **E** an INR (International Normalised Ratio) of less than 1 in a patient on warfarin therapy.

53 In a diabetic patient undergoing surgery:
- **A** on the day prior to surgery the dose of depot insulin should be halved and supplemented by soluble insulin later in the day.
- **B** half the normal daily insulin dose is given on the morning of surgery.
- **C** an intravenous infusion of 5% dextrose is erected on the morning of surgery.
- **D** if the blood sugar exceeds 11 mmol, one third of the daily insulin requirement may be given.
- **E** insulin requirements may increase after major surgery.

(Answers overleaf)

51 **A False** It may be prolonged due to malabsorption of vitamin K. Bile salts (absent from the intestine in obstructive jaundice) are necessary for the absorption of the fat soluble vitamins A, D, E and K.

B True The 'hepatorenal syndrome'.

C True This may have toxic effects on the kidney and contribute to renal dysfunction.

D False Jaundiced patients are often dehydrated, due to anorexia and hypodipsia. This may be compounded by vomiting. Measurement of serum electrolytes and adequate rehydration and resuscitation are essential before surgery is contemplated.

E True Probably due to suppression of the immune system.

52 **A True** Aspirin should be stopped for 5 days prior to surgery.

B False Protamine may be required to reverse the effects of heparin, which may increase bleeding during surgery.

C True This may be idiopathic or secondary to drug reactions, hypersplenism or disseminated intra-vascular coagulation (DIC).

D True Fibrinolysis may occur primarily in liver disease and metastatic carcinoma, or secondarily in the DIC syndrome.

E False When patients are anticoagulated with warfarin therapy, the INR is usually greater than 2.

53 **A True** To avoid hypoglycaemia on the day of surgery, due to the effects of long-acting insulin.

B False No insulin is given prior to surgery, as hypo-glycaemia is the major danger on the day of operation.

C True Again, to avoid hypoglycaemia on the day of operation.

D True But only once surgery has been completed.

E True Due to increased output of glucocorticoids which have an anti-insulin effect.

(For more information, see chs 10 and 11 of Principles and Practice of Surgery)

54 The following recommendations are appropriate in specific circumstances when a surgical procedure is contemplated:

A discontinuation of the contraceptive pill prior to elective surgery.

B administration of propranolol to a thyrotoxic patient.

C preferential use of regional anaesthesia in a patient with chronic chest disease.

D discontinuation of steroid drugs for 2 weeks prior to surgery.

E administration of 3 litres of fluid intravenously to jaundiced patients during the 24 hours prior to surgery.

55 In the immediate postoperative period:

A airway obstruction can occur following drug administration.

B airway obstruction results in hypoxia and hypercapnia.

C following total thyroidectomy, airway obstruction is prevented by closed suction drains.

D myocardial ischaemia presents with severe chest pain and is a straightforward clinical diagnosis.

E epidural anaesthesia can mask the signs of intra-abdominal haemorrhage.

56 Following major abdominal surgery:

A nasogastric suction prevents intestinal ileus.

B swinging pyrexia and diarrhoea are characteristic clinical features of a pelvic abscess.

C pulmonary atelectasis occurs frequently after laparoscopic cholecystectomy.

D open drainage reduces the risk of wound infection.

E small intestinal obstruction requires expeditious surgery to relieve this.

(Answers overleaf)

54 A False Current opinion favours continuing the contraceptive pill, as the risks of venous thrombosis associated with pregnancy outweigh those associated with an operation. Prophylaxis against thromboembolism is mandatory, however.

    B True 10–30 mg t.i.d. is used.

    C True To reduce the risks associated with general anaesthesia.

    D False Steroids should be continued to the time of surgery, and i.v. hydrocortisone should be administered in the perioperative period to avoid the risk of acute adrenocortical insufficiency, secondary to suppression of the pituitary–adrenal axis.

    E True To reduce dehydration and improve urine flow during the perioperative period.

55 A True Bronchospasm and full-blown anaphylaxis can occur as an idiosyncratic drug reaction. This may be very difficult to recognise in the unconscious patient.

    B True Airway obstruction results in type 2 respiratory failure and hypercapnia is a classical feature.

    C False Haemorrhage post-thyroidectomy is usually a sudden catastrophic event which suction drains will do little to correct.

    D False This is usually a silent event and is only apparent electrocardiographically or reflected by instability in the blood pressure and pulse.

    E True Hypotension may occur following epidural anaesthesia and the patient will not experience increasing peritonism associated with intra-abdominal haemorrhage.

56 A False Nasogastric suction is frequently employed to reduce the complications associated with postoperative ileus.

    B True Pelvic abscess classically presents in this fashion and most commonly occurs following a perforated appendix.

    C False The main advantage of laparoscopic cholecystectomy over open cholecystectomy is the decrease in pulmonary complications.

    D False Open drainage systems increase the risk of wound infection.

    E False As a general rule, small bowel obstruction should be alleviated within 24 hours of presentation. One exception is in the immediate postoperative period when adhesions are the main cause and usually settle spontaneously upon fasting and i.v. fluid replacement.

(For more information, see chs 10 and 11 of Principles and Practice of Surgery)

57 Postoperative pyrexia may occur secondary to:
A pulmonary atelectasis.
B deep venous thrombosis.
C subphrenic abscess.
D pulmonary embolism.
E blood transfusion.

58 Postoperatively:
A administration of non steroidal anti-inflammatory drugs can precipitate renal failure.
B deep venous thrombosis is reliably diagnosed if the lower limb is swollen, red and tender.
C pre-renal renal failure is corrected with intravenous diuretic administration.
D prolonged ileus and serosanguineous wound discharge suggests a wound infection.
E heparin prophylaxis prevents fatal pulmonary embolism.

59 The following are well recognised specific complications:
A positive Chevostek's sign after thyroid lobectomy.
B deep venous thrombosis after varicose vein surgery.
C hyponatraemia after craniotomy.
D cardiac dysrhythmia after total transthoracic oesophagectomy.
E urinary incontinence after inguinal hernia.

(Answers overleaf)

57 A True   Usually on the second postoperative day. The
                     problem is best resolved with aggressive physio-
                     therapy and adequate analgesia.

    B True   Low grade pyrexia on the sixth postoperative day
                     could well mean a DVT is present.

    C True   This is a serious infection with a mortality rate of
                     10–20%. Expeditious drainage is mandatory in
                     combination with intensive antibiotic therapy.

    D True   Although presentation may be catastrophic and fatal,
                     it may present in an indolent fashion with tachy-
                     pnoea, tachycardia and hypotension.

    E True   Pyrexia after or during blood transfusion is an
                     adverse sign and the transfusion should be aborted
                     and the blood checked for antibodies.

58 A True   NSAIDs are frequently employed in the postoperative
                     period. If the patient is hypovolaemic this can
                     precipitate renal failure. NSAIDs may also result in
                     acute renal failure secondary to papillary necrosis.

    B False   Clinical evaluation is very unreliable with a sensitivity
                     and specificity of approximately 50%. If one suspects
                     the diagnosis then a venogram should be performed.

    C False   Fluid replacement is the initial step.

    D False   This may be the predominant sign of abdominal
                     wound dehiscence.

    E False   To date, no single therapy has reduced the risk of
                     fatal pulmonary embolism.

59 A False   This, along with Trousseau's sign, is a feature of
                     hypocalcaemia. This would only be a worry after
                     subtotal or total thyroidectomy, where damage to all
                     parathyroids would be possible.

    B False   The incidence after varicose vein surgery is virtually
                     0%.

    C True   Due to inappropriate ADH release.

    D True   Atrial fibrillation is common after thoracotomy.

    E False   Urinary retention is much more common.

(For more information, see chs 10 and 11 of Principles and Practice of Surgery)

60 Potassium:

A is the major intracellular cation.
B concentrations are increased in actute tubular necrosis.
C depletion occurs in Addison's disease.
D is excreted preferentially to hydrogen ions in gastric outlet obstruction.
E loss occurs in high enterocutaneous fistulae.

(Answers overleaf)

60 A True
    B True   Renal failure results in decreased secretion of K^+.
    C False   Due to decreased levels of mineralocorticoids.
    D False   The body conserves K^+ at the expense of a
                    worsening metabolic alkalosis.
    E True   Small bowel secretions are high in potassium.

(For more information, see chs 10 and 11 of Principles and Practice of Surgery)

7. Wounds and wound healing

61 Following a primary incision:
- **A** the acute inflammatory response initiates the healing process.
- **B** fibroblasts migrate into the wound within 24 hours.
- **C** monocytes release inflammatory mediators integral to wound healing.
- **D** the acidotic milieu induces fibroblast migration from the wound edges.
- **E** collagen lysis is important in wound healing.

62 Two weeks following a primary incision:
- **A** polymorphonuclear cells are the predominant cell type at the healing interface.
- **B** neovascularisation is maximal.
- **C** epithelialisation is commencing.
- **D** the wound has recovered 80% of its original tensile strength.
- **E** fibroblasts will facilitate contraction of the wound margins.

63 Wound healing:
- **A** is slow in elderly patients.
- **B** is enhanced by ingestion of high-protein enteral supplementation.
- **C** is dependent upon normal systemic levels of ascorbic acid.
- **D** is impaired in patients with zinc deficiency.
- **E** occurs at a rate independent of the wound site.

(Answers overleaf)

61 A True In the 72-hour period following injury (lag phase), capillary permeability is increased, resulting in accumulation of a protein-rich exudate and inflammatory cells.

    B False Fibroblast migration occurs maximally in the 'incremental' or proliferative phase. Fibroblasts are integral to collagen synthesis and consequently wound tensile strength.

    C True Monocytes release specific interleukins and growth factors which are thought to contribute to wound healing both locally and systemically.

    D True The high lactate levels resulting from transient ischaemia in the wound induce fibroblast migration.

    E True Three weeks following injury, collagen breakdown approaches and may temporarily surpass synthesis. Lysis is important in clearing up excess collagen.

62 A False PMN cells appear in the wound within 24 hours and are integral to the acute inflammatory response.

    B True Angiogenesis factors are released by endothelial and mononuclear cells, and capillary buds form fragile arcades delivering the nutrients and oxygen necessary for collagen synthesis.

    C False Epithelial cells at the wound edge lose their adhesion and migrate until they meet epithelial cells from the other side. This is an early phenomenon.

    D False The wound will only have recovered 30% of its tensile strength. It takes 6 months for the wound to recover 80% of the original tensile stength.

    E True Special fibroblasts containing myofibrils pull the wound margins together, catalysing wound healing. This is distinct from contracture formation, which is abnormal wound healing.

63 A False Healing occurs at a normal rate in the elderly provided there are no concomitant debilitating or adverse factors.

    B True High-protein diets hasten the increase in wound tensile strength.

    C True Vitamin C is crucial for the hydoxylation of proline and lysine which is incorporated into tropocollagen which polymerises to form collagen. It is also important in the formation of normal basement membrane in new vessels.

    D True Many enzymes, such as DNA and RNA polymerase, are zinc dependent.

    E False Blood supply is extremely variable in different body sites. Ischaemia is an important factor in delayed wound healing.

(For more information, see ch 12 of Principles and Practice of Surgery)

64 Wound healing is impaired in patients with:
   A obstructive jaundice.
   B diabetes mellitus.
   C Cushing's syndrome.
   D chronic obstructive airways disease.
   E antithrombin III deficiency.

65 Principles of wound management include:
   A meticulous debridement of contaminated wounds.
   B antibiotic prophylaxis in potentially contaminated wounds.
   C early skin closure in clean wounds.
   D careful peroperative haemostasis.
   E delayed primary closure in contaminated wounds.

66 Wound infection rates:
   A can be reduced by careful skin preparation with antiseptic solutions.
   B can be reduced by shaving the operative site 24 hours prior to surgery.
   C can be reduced by minimising the preoperative hospital stay.
   D following colorectal surgery have been reduced to <2% with the use of prophylactic antibiotics.
   E Are approximately 10% in clean wounds.

(Answers overleaf)

64 A True   Jaundice may occur secondary to malignancy. Per se
it results in impaired nutrition, host immune dysfunction and increased wound infection.

    B True   Due to decreased cellular phagocytic capacity and
diminished neutrophil chemotaxis. Vascular
insufficiency occurs secondary to micro- and
macrovascular disease.

    C True   The inflammatory response, collagen synthesis and
resistance to sepsis are impaired.

    D True   These patients have diminished oxygen saturation.
    E False

65 A True   Foreign material increases the incidence of wound
sepsis.

    B True   This reduces wound infection rates in procedures
such as appendicectomy, cholecystectomy and
colectomy.

    C True   Early skin closure reduces the risk of wound
contamination and affords a better cosmetic result.

    D True   This reduces the incidence of wound haematoma.
Overzealous use of diathermy and excessive suture
material in the wound is detrimental.

    E True   In contaminated or potentially contaminated
wounds, delaying closure permits reappraisal of
the wound and assurance that infection is not
present prior to closure.

66 A True   Iodine and chlorhexidine significantly reduce the
population of Gram-positive cocci, the main
offenders in endogenous wound infection.

    B False   Shaving, if performed, should be performed
immediately prior to surgery, not the previous day,
which has been shown to increase wound infection
rate.

    C True   A prolonged preoperative stay increases the risk to
the patient of nosocomial infection.

    D False   Antibiotic prophylaxis along with colonic preparation
has reduced the incidence of wound infection from
30% to 5–10% in colorectal surgery.

    E False   The accepted level of wound sepsis in clean
operations is approximately 2%.

(For more information, see ch 12 of Principles and Practice of Surgery)

67 With respect to healing of specialised tissues:

A fracture healing following internal fixation is dependent on abundant callus formation.

B fractures with intra-articular extension are best managed by open reduction and internal fixation.

C following neurotmesis, the patient can expect spontaneous full neuronal recovery.

D following axonotmesis, primary suture of the nerve sheath is required to facilitate nerve recovery.

E following neuropraxia, neuronal recovery occurs after Wallerian degeneration and regrowth at a rate of 1 mm per day.

68 Successful healing of a colonic anastomosis:

A is facilitated by fastidious colonic purgation.

B is unlikely if the calibre of the respective resection limits are different.

C is promoted by the administration of prophylactic antibiotics.

D is dependent upon a good blood supply and tension-free anastomosis.

E is dependent upon accurate apposition of mucosa with nonabsorbable suture material.

69 Abdominal wound dehiscence:

A normally presents in the first week following surgery.

B occurs in less than 1% of patients.

C presents with profuse serosanguineous wound discharge and paralytic ileus.

D is always catastrophic and easily diagnosed.

E is more likely if the serum albumin is <25 g/dl.

(Answers overleaf)

67 **A** **False** Following internal fixation, the fracture heals by direct union with no callus formation.

B **True** It is ideal to have intra-articular fractures anatomically reduced and fixed to reduce the risk of osteoarthritis, e.g. bi-malleolar fractures of the ankle.

C **False** After neurotmesis, the nerve is completely divided and will require primary suture or nerve graft if any function is to be recovered.

D **False** After axonotmesis, the axonal sheaths are maintained and the nerve will recover spontaneously after a period of Wallerian degeneration.

E **False** This injury usually occurs after prolonged direct pressure on the nerve and full recovery can be expected within days.

68 **A** **True** Colonic preparation is essential prior to elective colonic surgery, and in the emergency colectomy where primary anastomosis is preferred, on-table colonic lavage is performed to decrease the risk of colonic leak.

B **False** The resection limits are frequently unequal, especially if the colon has been obstructed, but this has no effect on the healing process.

C **False** Antibiotic prophylaxis has no effect on colonic healing, but will decrease the risk of wound sepsis.

D **True** A basic principle in any form of wound healing.

E **False** The modern approach to intestinal anastomosis is to perform a single layer of submucosal seromuscular sutures, with absorbable materials.

69 **A** **False** It occurs classically on the 10th postoperative day.

B **True**

C **True**

D **False** The presentation may be occult with partial wound breakdown and delayed presentation with an incisional hernia.

E **True** Hypoalbuminaemia is a useful indicator of malnutrition and is associated with impaired wound healing and an increased incidence of wound dehiscence.

(For more information, see ch 12 of Principles and Practice of Surgery)

70 Concerning a traumatic wound:

A if penetrating, it is best explored under general anaesthetic.

B following debridement of foreign material and excision of devitalised tissue, the wound should be closed loosely.

C to the pretibial region in the elderly, skin apposition with suture material is desirable as early as possible.

D where there is significant skin loss, it should be covered with a full-thickness (Wolfe) skin graft.

E where the mechanism of injury is crush or degloving, early closure or grafting is the primary aim.

(Answers overleaf)

70 A True   Exploration is best carried out under general
anaesthetic as the superficial appearance of the
injury usually belies the extent of underlying
damage.

B False   Although wounds can be meticulously debrided, they
will still harbour microorganisms capable of wound
infection, therefore primary closure is inadvisable.

C False   Sutures will compromise the blood supply further,
particularly venous drainage. Steristrips and Visco-
paste bandages with low elevation are sufficient
to promote wound healing.

D False   Full-thickness skin grafts are not usually used in the
emergency situation as their chance of survival is
low. Where the primary aim is to obtain skin
coverage, split-skin grafts are a better option.

E False   The primary aim is to remove all the devitalised
tissue. The degree of tissue necrosis is not always
apparent initially and a second operation is
recommended before any attempt at closure or graft
application.

(For more information, see ch 12 of Principles and Practice of Surgery)

8. Burns

71 Concerning normal human skin:

A the epidermis consists of a layer of keratinised stratified squamous epithelium which is of uniform thickness in all body sites.

B the dermis has no epithelial component.

C it accounts for <5% of lean body mass.

D its area is between 1.5–1.9 m² in adults.

E it contains a high proportion of mast cells in the dermis.

72 Burn injuries:

A are categorised solely according to the percentage of body surface involved.

B carry higher mortality rates at the extremes of life.

C resulting in partial-thickness injury rarely require fluid resuscitation.

D resulting in full-thickness injury are painful and erythematous.

E to the head and neck have the highest mortality rates.

73 Local effects of burn injury include:

A decreased capillary permeability and impaired lymphatic drainage.

B red cell destruction.

C release of prostaglandins, kinins, histamine and cytokines which have both beneficial and detrimental effects.

D an insensible water loss of 15 ml/m² per hour.

E coagulative necrosis of the dermis.

(Answers overleaf)

71 A False   Skin thickness is very variable depending on the stress the particular site endures, e.g. the face compared with the sole of the foot.

B False   The major skin adnexae are situated in the dermis, namely the hair follicles, sebaceous and sweat glands. These are lined with epithelial cells which are capable of reconstituting the normal surface epithelium after a burn and skin grafting.

C False   Skin is one of the largest organs, constituting 15% of lean body mass.

D True

E True   Mast cells are prominent at the internal–external body interface so that they can react with foreign allergens. They are predominant in the dermis and are responsible for IgE-mediated type I hypersensitivity reactions resulting in urticaria.

72 A False   Although the percentage burn is the most important parameter, the depth of the burn is also significant in future management and outcome.

B True   Young adults tolerate burns better than the very young or the elderly.

C False   Superficial burns are just as likely to incur major fluid and electrolyte disturbances as full-thickness burns.

D False   Full-thickness burns destroy the cutaneous nerve endings and have a dead white appearance on account of destruction of the dermal capillaries.

E True   These burn injuries are more frequently associated with concomitant smoke inhalation and a wide variety of respiratory insults, which significantly affect the morbidity and mortality from burns.

73 A False   Capillary permeability is increased within minutes of the burn. Plasma exuded into the interstitial space overwhelms the lymphatic drainage and is maximal in the first 24 hours, but usually returns to normal by 48 hours.

B True   Full-thickness burns will result in red cell destruction.

C True   These contribute to the formation of tissue oedema and may augment host immune function. Their effects on the microcirculation locally and systemically may increase the burn depth over the initial 48 hours and may result in systemic organ dysfunction.

D False   This is the normal insensible loss. Following a burn this can increase to up to 200 ml/m^2 per hour.

E True   The epidermis and dermis are converted into the eschar by way of coagulative necrosis. If left, this will separate and slough spontaneously after 3 weeks, leaving a healthy bed of granulation tissue.

(For more information, see ch 13 of Principles and Practice of Surgery)

74 The general effects of burn injury:
   A are independent of the size of the burn area.
   B include immune suppression.
   C result in decreased urinary nitrogen concentrations.
   D include hypoalbuminaemia.
   E include hyponatraemia.

75 The following are useful determinants of burn depth:
   A the nature of the injurious insult.
   B intact cutaneous sensation.
   C the presence or absence of erythema.
   D blister formation.
   E the degree of fluid loss from the burn surface.

76 The risks to the burn victim include:
   A intrinsic renal failure.
   B cerebral oedema.
   C peptic ulceration.
   D nosocomial pneumonia.
   E heterotopic calcification.

(Answers overleaf)

74 A False The larger the burn area the greater the systemic insult.

B True In large burns, both humoral and cellular immune function are depressed.

C False The metabolic response to trauma results in marked gluconeogenesis and considerable urinary nitrogen loss.

D True Due to local loss from the burn and impaired liver synthesis.

E True There is loss from the burn oedema, failure of the cellular sodium pump and marked ADH secretion following the burn. This can be sufficiently severe to produce convulsions and fatal cerebral oedema.

75 A True Scalds and flash burns are usually partial-thickness, whereas contact burns and electrical burns are invariably full-thickness.

B True Intact sensation infers a superficial injury.

C True Deep burns are usually white or leathery brown due to eschar formation. Partial-thickness burns are erythematous and blanch on pressure.

D True A feature of partial-thickness injury.

E False Even partial-thickness burns will result in marked fluid loss. The most important determinant of fluid loss is the extent rather than the depth of the burn.

76 A True Intrinsic failure can still occur from prolonged hypovolaemia, haemoglobinuria, myoglobinuria and endotoxaemia resulting from local or generalised sepsis.

B True From the hyponatraemia and fluid retention secondary to ADH secretion.

C True Curling's ulcers are well recognised after burn injury.

D True Prolonged hospitalisation, immune suppression and bacterial translocation increase the risk of hospital-acquired respiratory infection.

E True

(For more information, see ch 13 of Principles and Practice of Surgery)

77 Immediate management of the severely burned patient includes:

   A intravenous plasma administration of 0.5–0.65 ml/kg body weight per % burn in the 4-hour period from the time of injury.
   B blood transfusion.
   C administration of tetanus toxoid.
   D insertion of a urinary catheter and hourly urometer.
   E avoidance of opiate analgesia which will suppress respiratory function.

78 In the early local management of burns:

   A superficial burns should never be left exposed to the atmosphere.
   B wounds should be meticulously cleansed and devitalised tissue excised.
   C partial-thickness burns will require early split-skin grafting.
   D broad-spectrum antibiotics should be administered.
   E dressings should be occlusive, nonabsorptive and changed on a daily basis.

79 In the management of deep burns:

   A early tangential excision of the eschar and skin grafting are recommended.
   B escharotomy for circumferential burns is advisable.
   C eschar should be left intact as this reduces the risk of secondary infection.
   D to the neck, expeditious grafting and splinting should be performed to avoid serious flexion contractures.
   E of greater than 20%, blood transfusion is required.

(Answers overleaf)

77 A True   Fluid requirement (ml) is calculated from patient weight (kg) x % burn divided by 2. The first 36 hours post-surgery are divided into six successive periods of time (4,4,4,6,6 and 12 hours) and the calculated volume of fluid should be administered in each time quantum.

B False   Blood loss occurs at a rate of approximately 1% volume for every 1% full-thickness burn. This is not a consideration unless the burn area exceeds 10%, and is not an immediate consideration in the initial resuscitation period.

C True

D True   This will give an accurate measurement of hourly urine production and permits titration of intravenous fluids in the initial period of intravascular resuscitation.

E False   Opiate analgesics are routinely employed and form part of the mainstay of early management in burned patients.

78 A False   Facial burns and burns which involve one surface may be left exposed.

B True   As with any contaminated wound, debridement is the gold standard.

C False   Partial-thickness burns will heal spontaneously, usually within 3 weeks.

D False   This will increase antibiotic-resistant bacterial strains, and application of dressings with bactericidal creams forms the mainstay of treatment. Antibiotics are reserved for overwhelming life-threatening sepsis.

E False   Ideally, dressings should absorb wound exudate only necessitating change if the exudate threatens to soak through. Repetitive dressings remove fragile new epithelium and increase the risk of sepsis.

79 A True   This practice saves time in hospital, reducing overall cost and reducing the sepsis-related morbidity and mortality for the patient.

B True   This is mandatory, as this form of burn will result in compression and vascular compromise of the respective extremity or restriction of chest expansion.

C False   Eschar is not impervious to bacteria; indeed, pseudomonas species and some Gram-negative bacteria release enzymes which hasten separation of the eschar.

D True   This is a common site for early contracture formation. It can quickly present problems if tracheostomy is required for future airway management.

E True   Usually burns of >10% will require transfusion. This percentage is less in children.

(For more information, see ch 13 of Principles and Practice of Surgery)

80 Modern management of burned patients includes:

A early institution of enteral feeding.

B antibiotic therapy aimed at sterilising the burn site prior to grafting.

C meshing of split-skin grafts which can provide up to six times the potential coverage of the graft.

D pressure dressings and splints to reduce contracture formation.

E early release of contractures to provide the best functional and aesthetic result.

(Answers overleaf)

80 A True   Enteral feeding will offset the severe protein loss occurring as a result of the metabolic response to the burn and decrease the risk of systemic sepsis and multiple organ dysfunction.

    B False   This breeds opportunistic infections with yeasts, fungi and resistant strains of bacteria. It is impossible to sterilise the site prior to grafting. By use of dressings such as silver nitrate soaks or silver sulphadiazine, the incidence of *Pseudomonas aeruginosa* colonisation is greatly reduced. Early infection of a burn wound with β haemolytic streptococcus (*Strep. pyogenes*) is a potential disaster. Where the risks of this are high, e.g. a child with a sore throat, then prophylactic penicillin or erythromycin can be usefully employed.

    C True

    D True   Hypertrophic scar formation is due to an imbalance in the reparative and regenerative process. Early splinting, pressure dressings and physiotherapy are important in achieving the best functional result following burn injury.

    E False   Premature surgical intervention before contracture maturation increases the number of procedures required and results in a worse aesthetic result.

(For more information, see ch 13 of Principles and Practice of Surgery)

9. Trauma and multiple injury

81 Concerning trauma:
- **A** it is the commonest cause of death between the ages of 1 week and 45 years.
- **B** it may be due to a low velocity missile fired from a machine gun or rifle.
- **C** high velocity missiles produce more extensive damage than low velocity missiles.
- **D** blast injury is due to a combination of low and high velocity missiles only.
- **E** road traffic accidents are the most common cause of blunt injury.

82 With respect to trauma assessment and resuscitation:
- **A** it involves a formalised approach in the initial stage which is the same for every patient.
- **B** the primary survey involves assessment of gastrointestinal and urological injuries.
- **C** the secondary survey commences before the resuscitation phase.
- **D** hyperextension of the neck may help secure the airway.
- **E** oxygen therapy should be instituted for all trauma patients.

83 Concerning trauma assessment and resuscitation:
- **A** exsanguination of the blood volume by 25% results in unconsciousness.
- **B** skin perfusion is maintained until blood loss reaches 40% of the total blood volume.
- **C** carotid and femoral pulses are usually lost when the blood volume is depleted by 30%.
- **D** tourniquets are very useful to control limb haemorrhage.
- **E** vasopressors, steroids and sodium bicarbonate are useful in treating hypovolaemic shock.

(Answers overleaf)

81 A True

   B False Low velocity missiles are fired from handguns; rifles or machine guns fire high velocity missiles (>1000 m/s).

   C True Due to greater amount of energy (kinetic energy = $\frac{mv^2}{2}$) being transferred to the tissues (high energy transfer) with resultant compression and acceleration of tissue away from the bullet tract (cavitation).

   D False It is due to these (shrapnel and flying debris) plus the blast shock wave, an air wave which travels at just over the speed of sound.

   E True Stab and firearm injuries represent the most common cause of penetrating injury.

82 A True This is the *primary survey*, involving (a) airway and cervical spine control, (b) breathing, (c) circulation, (d) disability (neurological assessment), (e) exposure (ensuring that the patient is fully exposed to allow complete examination).

   B False The primary survey deals with immediate, life-threatening injuries (e.g. airway obstruction, exsanguinating haemorrhage). Assessment of other injuries (e.g. urological) is carried out in the *secondary survey*.

   C False The secondary survey does not commence until the primary survey has been completed and the resuscitation phase has begun.

   D False Hyperextension of the neck may exacerbate a cervical injury and should not be performed.

   E True Via a face mask — nasal prongs do not achieve a sufficient FiO_2.

83 A False Unconsciousness results when the blood volume is reduced by 50% or more.

   B False In hypovolaemia, blood is diverted away from the skin and peripheries — ashen facial and white skin appearances usually indicate blood loss of at least 30%.

   C False These are usually palpable until blood loss reaches 50%.

   D False Tourniquets should not be used as they can result in anaerobic metabolism. They can also increase blood loss if applied incorrectly. Local compression should be used to control haemorrhage.

   E False These should not be used. The treatment of hypovolaemic shock involves fluid and blood replacement.

(For more information, see ch 14 of Principles and Practice of Surgery)

84 Concerning trauma assessment and resuscitation:

A it involves early insertion of two large-calibre (>16 gauge) intravenous catheters.

B it involves early insertion of a urinary catheter in all patients.

C ECG monitoring of all trauma victims should be performed.

D a nasogastric tube should be inserted in all patients.

E neurological assessment usually takes several minutes.

85 Appropriate X-ray investigations in a multiple trauma victim include:

A an early skull X-ray to exclude a skull fracture.

B an early cervical spine X-ray to exclude a fracture.

C a chest X-ray.

D an abdominal X-ray.

E an X-ray of the pelvis.

86 Concerning thoracic injury:

A a simple pneumothorax should be treated by insertion of an intercostal drain in the 3rd interspace, mid-clavicular line.

B an intercostal drain should be inserted using a trocar to direct it towards the apex of the pleural cavity.

C rupture of the diaphragm usually occurs on the left side.

D subcutaneous emphysema requires immediate needle insertion and drainage.

E flail chest occurs when more than one rib is fractured.

(Answers overleaf)

84 **A True**   Usually in each antecubital fossa.
    B False   A urinary catheter should not be inserted if there is blood at the external meatus or in the scrotum, or if the prostate cannot be palpated on rectal examination (these are all signs of a possible membranous urethral injury).
    C True   This may detect arrhythmias due to cardiac contusion, hypothermia, hypoperfusion or hypoxia.
    D False   In patients with multiple or head trauma, a fracture of the cribriform plate must be excluded by X-ray, prior to nasogastric tube insertion. Attempted insertion in the presence of such a fracture can result in the tube entering the cranial cavity.
    E False   This can be rapidly performed using the AVPU method: A = alert, V = responds to vocal command, P = responds to painful stimuli, U = unresponsive. For more accurate follow-up and monitoring, the Glasgow Coma Scale is used.

85 **A False**   The presence or absence of a skull fracture does not alter the early assessment and resuscitation.
    B True   An unstable cervical spine must be recognised early and protected.
    C True   To detect a potentially life-threatening injury such as a pneumothorax (which can be missed clinically), or an aortic rupture (indicated by widening of the mediastinum).
    D False   This does not provide any information which alters the initial assessment and resuscitation.
    E True   It is important to detect a pelvic fracture as this indicates significant force to the body and can result in substantial blood loss. The three most important early radiological investigations, therefore, are X-rays of the cervical spine, chest and pelvis.

86 **A False**   It should be inserted laterally — in the 5th or 6th interspace, mid-axillary line.
    B False   It should be inserted using a blunt technique, which involves dissection over the rib and insertion of a finger into the pleural cavity, prior to insertion of the drain.
    C True   On the right it is relatively well protected by the liver.
    D False   Subcutaneous emphysema is usually absorbed — it does not require treatment.
    E False   It occurs when one or more ribs are fractured in two places, resulting in an isolated segment of the chest wall which moves paradoxically with respiration.

(For more information, see ch 14 of Principles and Practice of Surgery)

87 In thoracic trauma:

   A a tension pneumothorax should be treated initially by immediate needle thoracentesis on that side.

   B widening of the mediastinum on a chest X-ray may suggest a rupture of the aorta.

   C blunt injury to the chest may be associated with an elevation of the myocardial enzymes.

   D the upper ribs (1–3) are those most commonly fractured in blunt injuries.

   E a haemothorax requires early thoracotomy.

88 In abdominal trauma:

   A the presence of blood in the peritoneal cavity may be reliably detected by a generalised 'white' appearance on an abdominal radiograph.

   B diagnostic peritoneal lavage (DPL) should be performed in all cases of penetrating abdominal trauma.

   C the liver is the organ most often damaged by blunt trauma.

   D penetrating abdominal wounds are always managed by exploratory laparotomy.

   E blood loss from a pelvic fracture is usually self-limiting and causes little haemodynamic upset.

89 Concerning the multiple trauma patient:

   A immediate assessment and reduction of extremity fractures is the first priority.

   B patients with compound fractures should be given antibiotics.

   C a rectal examination is mandatory in all patients.

   D signs of cardiac tamponade include hypotension, neck vein distension and increased heart sounds.

   E cardiac tamponade should be treated by pericardiocentesis, which involves insertion, of an aspirating needle in the area of the apex beat.

(Answers overleaf)

87 **A** **True**   This may help improve cardiovascular and
                respiratory function by decompressing that side of
                the chest; an intercostal drain can then be inserted.
    B **True**
    C **True**   Due to myocardial contusion.
    D **False**   The middle ribs (4–9) sustain the majority of blunt
                trauma.
    E **False**   In the vast majority of cases, a haemothorax is
                caused by lung laceration or laceration of an
                intercostal vessel or internal mammary artery.
                Bleeding due to this is usually self-limiting, and
                operative intervention (apart from insertion of an
                intercostal drain) is not required.

88 **A** **False**   Plain X-rays are of limited value in detecting
                abdominal injury. The presence of blood is best
                detected by diagnostic peritoneal lavage.
    B **False**   DPL is most frequently used for detection of injury
                following blunt abdominal trauma. In most cases of
                penetrating abdominal trauma (particularly gunshot
                wounds) exploratory laparotomy is indicated.
    C **False**   The spleen is most often damaged.
    D **False**   This is true for gunshot wounds. In stab wounds, the
                wound can be explored under local anaesthetic to
                see if the peritoneum has been breached. If not,
                laparotomy is not required.
    E **False**   Blood loss from a pelvic fracture can be excessive —
                up to 4 or 5 litres.

89 **A** **False**   Immediate assessment and management in the
                primary survey (ABCDE) is the first priority.
    B **True**
    C **True**   To assess sphincter tone (which may be lost in spinal
                injuries) and the position of the prostate (which may
                be high if there is a rupture of the urethra).
    D **False**   Signs of cardiac tamponade include hypotension,
                neck vein distension and 'muffled' or 'distant' heart
                sounds (Beck's triad).
    E **False**   The aspirating needle is inserted in the subxyphoid
                area with the needle angled at 45° left of the midline
                and 45° above the chest wall.

(For more information, see ch 14 of Principles and Practice of Surgery)

90 Concerning multiple trauma:

A lung complications may develop even though there has been no significant thoracic trauma.

B insertion of a jejunal feeding tube is recommended.

C restlessness and uncooperative behaviour suggest that the patient has a significant head injury.

D skull fractures are usually associated with significant neurological injury.

E the presence of bruising or ecchymosis in the mastoid region indicates the possibility of a basal skull fracture.

(Answers overleaf)

90 A True   This is known as the adult respiratory distress
                   syndrome (ARDS) — thought to occur secondary to
                   release of cytokines and other products following
                   tissue trauma or sepsis.

    B True   This allows enteral feeding in the immediate and
                   later postoperative periods and avoids the
                   complications and expense of parenteral nutrition
                   (e.g. line sepsis, pneumothorax, venous thrombosis).

    C False   This suggests that the patient is hypoxic.

    D False   The majority of patients with skull fractures have
                   minimal neurological deficit. The significance of a
                   skull fracture is that it identifies the patient with
                   a higher probability of having, or developing, an
                   intracranial haematoma.

    E True   Battle's sign.

(For more information, see ch 14 of Principles and Practice of Surgery)

10. Organ transplantation

91 United Kingdom requirements for diagnosis of brain stem death prior to organ procurement include the following:

A the patient is unresponsive and on a ventilator.
B the cause of coma has been properly ascertained.
C exclusion of causes of potentially reversible apnoeic coma.
D exclusion of malignant disease as a cause of coma.
E assessment of all criteria by three doctors.

92 Loss of brain stem function is ascertained by establishing the absence of the following brain stem reflexes:

A pupillary response to light.
B corneal reflex.
C vestibulo-ocular reflex (caloric test).
D gag reflex.
E persistence of apnoea in the presence of a P_{CO_2} above 6.65 kPa.

93 Indications for renal transplantation include:

A polycystic disease.
B trauma.
C acute pyelonephritis.
D chronic glomerulonephritis.
E renal cell carcinoma.

94 Renal transplantation:

A in the majority of cases involves a live related donor.
B in the majority of cases involves a live unrelated donor.
C involves placement of the transplanted kidney in the site of one of the recipient's kidneys.
D may be performed if a kidney has been stored with a cold ischaemia time of up to 5 days.
E may only be performed on one occasion because of severe host-versus-graft response if a second transplantation is attempted.

(Answers overleaf)

91 A True
    B True
    C True   Examples include drugs which depress the CNS, and metabolic or endocrine disturbances.
    D False   The presence of malignant disease is usually a contraindication to organ procurement for transplantation. Exclusion of it is not a requirement for diagnosing brain stem death.
    E False   This has to be done by two doctors.

92 A True
    B True
    C True   Tested by flushing the external auditory canal with ice cold water.
    D True   Tested as part of the overall motor response within the cranial nerve distribution.
    E True   This level is sufficient to stimulate the respiratory centre if it is alive.

93 A True
    B True   Although it is rare for both kidneys to be lost due to trauma. Before performing a nephrectomy in a trauma case it is essential to ascertain that a contralateral functioning kidney is present.
    C False   Chronic pyelonephritis (e.g. due to chronic vesicoureteric reflux) is a common cause of renal failure and indication for transplantation.
    D True
    E False   The treatment for this includes surgical resection and adjuvant therapy (e.g. with interferon), but not transplantation.

94 A False
    B False   Approximately 95% of transplanted kidneys come from cadaveric donors.
    C False   It is placed extraperitoneally in the iliac fossa and is vascularised from the iliac vessels. The ureter is implanted directly into the bladder.
    D False   The maximum is approximately 72 hours, but implantation should preferably occur after a cold ischaemia time much shorter than this.
    E False   Retransplantation is feasible if a first graft fails whether due to rejection, technical or other problems.

(For more information, see ch 15 of Principles and Practice of Surgery)

95 Side effects and risks of immunosuppressive therapy include:

A gingival hypertrophy.
B loss of body hair.
C infection.
D development of neoplasia.
E osteoporosis.

96 Concerning transplantation:

A blood transfusion is an example of cellular transplantation.
B bone transplantation is an example of organ transplantation.
C pancreas transplantation is an example of solid organ transplantation.
D bone marrow transplantation is an example of organ transplantation.
E liver transplantation is an example of tissue transplantation.

97 Liver transplantation:

A requires HLA tissue typing as well as ABO and rhesus blood group matching if it is to be successful.
B may be successful if a noncompatible liver in terms of ABO grouping is used.
C may be performed between a living donor and a related recipient.
D is commonly performed for secondary malignant disease of the liver.
E is associated with chronic graft rejection in up to 40% of cases.

98 Pancreas transplantation:

A is generally performed for exocrine insufficiency.
B is as widely used and successful as renal or liver transplantation.
C may involve solid organ or cellular transplantation.
D is often performed in association with kidney transplantation.
E is associated with a one-year patient survival of 60%.

(Answers overleaf)

95 A True   Particularly with cyclosporin A.
  B False   Hirsutism is a problem with cyclosporin A and steroids.
  C True   Particularly frequent are fungal infections and viral infections such as herpes and cytomegalovirus.
  D True   Particularly skin cancers and lymphoid tumours.
  E True   Particularly with steroids.

96 A True
  B False   Tissue transplantation — in this case it is the noncellular matrix which is important, providing a framework into which recipient cells may grow.
  C True   Pancreatic islet transplantation is also an example of cellular transplantation.
  D False   Cellular transplantation.
  E False   Solid organ transplantation.

97 A False   Only ABO and rhesus group matching is routinely performed.
  B True   In extreme emergencies, where no other liver is available, this may be performed (e.g. acute hepatic coma due to hepatitis).
  C True   By resecting part of the donor's liver, e.g. segments II and III, and transplanting it into a small recipient (e.g. young child).
  D False   Results in this situation are extremely poor — it is most commonly performed for primary parenchymal disorders (e.g. cirrhosis).
  E False   This occurs in up to 10% of cases.

98 A False   For endocrine insufficiency (diabetes mellitus).
  B False   Technical and rejection problems mean that results for this are not as good as for kidney or liver transplantation.
  C True   Both solid pancreas and islet transplantation are used.
  D True   In diabetic patients who have developed secondary renovascular disease and renal failure.
  E False   One-year survival is currently 90%, with 75% of patients remaining insulin-independent.

(For more information, see ch 15 of Principles and Practice of Surgery)

99 Heart transplantation:
   A is indicated for ischaemic heart disease.
   B is indicated for selected cases of congenital heart disease.
   C is contraindicated in patients with cardiomyopathy.
   D is contraindicated in pulmonary hypertension.
   E may be combined with lung transplantation.

100 Concerning transplantation:
   A small bowel transplantation has not been successfully
         performed.
   B it is not possible to perform transplantation of more than
         two abdominal organs.
   C in most countries, the cadaveric donation pool is sufficient
         to meet requirements.
   D liver transplantation is contraindicated in cases of alcoholic
         cirrhosis.
   E living related organ donation is being performed
         increasingly frequently.

(Answers overleaf)

99　**A**　**True**

　　　B　**True**

　　　C　**False**　This is one of the major indications.

　　　D　**True**

　　　E　**True**　For example, in cases of pulmonary hypertension, Eisenmenger's complex, cystic fibrosis and emphysema.

100　**A**　**False**　But results, in terms of survival, are as yet very poor.

　　　B　**False**　Patients have survived after 'cluster' transplantation of multiple organs including liver, pancreas, stomach and intestine.

　　　C　**False**　Requirements excessively outweigh availability of cadaveric organs.

　　　D　**False**　But patients must have stopped drinking and demonstrated abstinence over a prolonged period (e.g. 6–12 months).

　　　E　**True**　Due to the shortage of cadaveric donors and the fact that in some countries (e.g. Japan) cadaveric donation is prohibited.

(For more information, see ch 15 of Principles and Practice of Surgery)

11. Principles of surgery for cancer

101 **The following are recognised induction agents in carcinogenesis:**
- **A** retrovirus infection.
- **B** nitrosamines.
- **C** coal tar.
- **D** ultra violet light.
- **E** malnutrition.

102 **The following factors can directly influence tumour behaviour:**
- **A** immunocompetence of the host.
- **B** infection with the Epstein–Barr virus.
- **C** age.
- **D** gender.
- **E** p53 allele expression.

(Answers overleaf)

101 A True   This represents the pathophysiological mechanism of viral oncogenesis. Integration of a nondefective retrovirus in close proximity to the proto-oncogene results in a detrimental qualitative and/or quantitative expression of the oncogene with neoplastic transformation.

    B True   As food preservatives they have been implicated in the development of colonic carcinoma.

    C True   This contains a variety of hydrocarbons capable of inducing tumorigenesis, e.g. bronchogenic carcinoma from cigarette smoking, Potts' scrotal carcinoma in chimney sweeps.

    D True   Radiation can result in alteration of normal DNA, which is the primary insult in carcinogenesis.

    E False   Quite the converse. Those who are >25% overweight have a greater incidence of carcinoma of the endometrium, breast, colon and pancreas.

102 A True   Immune status both directly affects the host's ability to combat the neoplasm, and influences the risk of tumour development, e.g. Kaposi sarcoma in AIDS.

    B True   This virus is fascinating with respect to its effects in different races. It is associated with the development of Burkitt's lymphoma in children living in the African subcontinent, and nasopharyngeal carcinoma in the Far East.

    C False   Although neoplasms occur more frequently with increasing age there is no direct relationship between age and the behaviour of a tumour.

    D False   Hormone status has a potent effect on tumours specific to an individual's gender, e.g. prostate; however, the sex of the individual has no effect on the tumour's behaviour.

    E True   This is a tumour-suppressor gene which if deficient or present in the mutant form will result in an increase in tumour formation.

(For more information, see ch 16 of Principles and Practice of Surgery)

103   The following features differentiate between benign and malignant neoplasms:

A   capacity of the tumour to invade neighbouring tissues.
B   ulceration of the overlying skin.
C   capacity of the tumour to metastasise to remote sites.
D   dysplastic nature of the cells constituting the tumour.
E   capacity of the tumour to secrete hormones.

104   The growth of the following tumours is hormone dependent:

A   lobular carcinoma of the breast.
B   follicular carcinoma of the thyroid.
C   prostatic carcinoma.
D   small cell anaplastic tumour of the lung.
E   endometrial leiomyosarcoma.

105   Ionising radiation may give rise to the following malignancies:

A   leukaemia.
B   thyroid malignancy.
C   teratoma of the ovary.
D   osteogenic sarcoma.
E   colonic carcinoma.

(Answers overleaf)

103 A True   The main primary feature of any malignancy is its ability to destroy natural barriers such as organ capsules and basement membranes.

B False   Large benign neoplasms can undergo ischaemic necrosis and ulcerate, and if sufficiently large may ulcerate through overlying structures, e.g. cystosarcoma phylloides tumour of the breast, leiomyoma of the uterus.

C True   This characteristic is exclusive to malignant tumours.

D False   Cells may be dysplastic without being frankly malignant. Normally there is a sequential progression from dysplasia to malignant transformation.

E False   Both benign and malignant tumours have the potential for hormone release. Some malignant tumours have inappropriate hormone release resulting in an array of paraneoplastic syndromes.

104 A True   Breast carcinomata frequently express oestrogen receptors and it has been shown that adjuvant hormonal manipulation targetted at reducing oestrogen levels will improve survival in patients with breast cancer.

B True   This tumour will respond to thyroxine therapy, although this is not the treatment of choice.

C True   Stilboestrol therapy is still employed in this condition although more novel methods are now available, namely LHRH antagonists and androgen blockade.

D False   This tumour may secrete a variety of hormones but is not hormone dependent per se.

E False   Widespread endometrial carcinoma is treated by progestogen therapy; however, sarcomas do not respond to hormonal manipulation.

105 A True   This is one of the commonest malignancies (along with squamous carcinoma of skin) associated with ionising radiation.

B True   This is well recognised, and personnel exposed regularly to ionising radiation, e.g. radiographers, radiologists, dentists, should routinely wear a coat with a protective lead collar.

C False   Infertility is the main concern here. There is no evidence to suggest that ionising radiation increases the risk of malignancy.

D True
E False

(For more information, see ch 16 of Principles and Practice of Surgery)

106 The following tumours exhibit characteristic metastatic potential:

A papillary carcinoma of the thyroid — early blood-borne dissemination.

B osteogenic sarcoma — early spread to para-aortic lymph nodes.

C rectal carcinoma — early dissemination to liver parenchyma.

D cerebral astrocytoma — blood-borne spread to bone and lung.

E papillary carcinoma of the ovary — local spread to the peritoneal cavity.

107 The following statements are true:

A renal carcinoma may give rise to inferior vena cava obstruction.

B neoplasms of the caecum and ascending colon frequently present with intestinal obstruction.

C lymphoma of the thyroid gland is a late complication of Hashimoto's thyroiditis.

D bronchogenic carcinoma may produce hypernatraemia.

E gastric carcinoma may metastasise to the ovary.

(Answers overleaf)

106 **A** **False** This tumour classically presents in the young, spreads to local cervical lymph nodes (NB lateral aberrant thyroid) and has an excellent prognosis.

   B **False** This highly aggressive neoplasm usually presents in the second decade of life around the metaphysis of long bones and disseminates early in its course to the lung.

   C **False** Rectal tumours, as with other colonic neoplasms, normally spread to regional lymph nodes before ultimately metastasising to the liver.

   D **False** Primary brain tumours characteristically do not metastasise extracranially.

   E **True** This describes transcoelomic spread, which is characteristic of ovarian tumours.

107 **A** **True** Renal carcinomata frequently spread to the renal vein, and the tumour may obstruct the IVC.

   B **False** These tumours present occultly with alternating bowel pattern and anaemia. Tumours of the left colon present overtly with intestinal obstruction and painless rectal bleeding.

   C **True**

   D **False** Bronchogenic neoplasms may secrete antidiuretic hormone which results in hyponatraemia.

   E **True** This is well recognised and is known as a Krükenberg tumour. It can also occur from a primary tumour in the colon or breast.

(For more information, see ch 16 of Principles and Practice of Surgery)

108 Screening has been successfully employed in early detection of the following tumours:

 A cervical carcinoma.
 B breast carcinoma.
 C colonic carcinoma.
 D pancreatic carcinoma.
 E ovarian carcinoma.

109 These tumours secrete the following specific tumour markers:

 A prostatic carcinoma — prostate specific antigen..
 B testicular seminoma — human chorionic gonadotrophin.
 C ovarian carcinoma — CA125.
 D cholangiocarcinoma — alphafetoprotein.
 E colonic carcinoma — carcinoembryonic antigen (CEA).

(Answers overleaf)

108 **A** **True** Early detection of dysplastic cervical epithelium identifies women at risk of developing frank malignancy. This permits surgical intervention at an opportune time to abort malignant transformation.

B **True** Presently, women in the UK over the age of 50 should undergo mammography every 3–5 years, which will diagnose with 95% sensitivity early impalpable breast tumours. There is some contention as to whether this will ultimately improve patient survival.

C **False** Selective screening of individuals with faecal occult blood and sigmoidoscopy has been employed in some countries but is not universally practised.

D **False** For any screening method to be employed efficaciously it must be applied in a common disease, where there is a simple, economic, non-invasive, sensitive and specific test which will allow early treatment to be implemented to improve survival statistics. This is unrealistic in pancreatic cancer.

E **False** Nevertheless, ubiquitous availability of ultra-sonography and sensitive serum tumour markers may increase the possibility of this becoming useful.

109 **A** **True**

B **False** Pure seminomas do not secrete HCG or alphafetoprotein; however, if the tumour has teratomatous elements then these tumour-specific antigens may be expressed.

C **True**

D **False** Hepatocellular carcinomata express this specific tumour marker. Cholangiocarcinoma does not express any specific marker.

E **True** Many tumours express this antigen. Colorectal carcinoma is the best recognised; however, cancers of breast, liver, bronchus and pancreas will all express this antigen to a greater or lesser extent.

(For more information, see ch 16 of Principles and Practice of Surgery)

110 The following treatment modalities are usefully employed in the following malignant diseases:

A systemic delivery of cyclophosphamide, methotrexate and 5-fluorouracil as adjuvant therapy for stage II breast carcinoma in premenopausal women.

B external beam radiotherapy as first-line management for squamous carcinoma of the anus.

C prophylactic block dissection of regional lymph nodes in malignant melanoma.

D external beam radiotherapy to para-aortic lymph nodes in stage I teratoma.

E adjuvant systemic 5-fluorouracil for Duke's B and C colo-rectal carcinoma.

(Answers overleaf)

110 **A True**   This is the Bonnadonna regiment which has demonstrated an 8% increased survival in this patient population.

     B True   This is the gold standard approach to anal carcinoma and has superseded abdominoperineal resection of the rectum in most centres.

     C False   This is no longer employed unless the regional lymph nodes are involved with the tumour.

     D False   Stage I teratomas do not require any adjuvant therapy and should be managed with rigorous clinical, serological and radiological review. Stage I seminomas should have prophylactic radiotherapy to para-aortic glands.

     E True   This is widely employed now but initially found favour in the USA.

(For more information, see ch 16 of Principles and Practice of Surgery)

12. Skin, connective tissue and soft tissues

111 **The following are features of a sebaceous cyst:**
- **A** it arises in the epidermis.
- **B** it has a central punctum.
- **C** it contains degenerative mucopolysaccharides.
- **D** it demonstrates fluctuance.
- **E** it occurs commonly on the scalp.

112 **Dermoid cysts:**
- **A** arise from the sequestration of epidermal cells within the dermis.
- **B** occur exclusively as a congenital phenomenon.
- **C** occur in the suprasternal space of Burns.
- **D** contain sebum.
- **E** are superficial and suitable for excision under local anaesthetic.

113 **The following are premalignant conditions:**
- **A** actinic keratoses.
- **B** Bowen's disease.
- **C** erythroplasia of De Queyrat.
- **D** tylosis.
- **E** giant hairy naevus.

(Answers overleaf)

111 A False It arises in the dermis and skin can normally be moved over it.

B True

C False This is the content of a ganglion. Sebaceous cysts contain sebum.

D False Although cystic, this sign is difficult to demonstrate and is more classically demonstrable in a lipoma.

E True This is a common site and sebaceous cysts are frequently multiple.

112 A True

B False Although they arise as congenital anomalies at the sites of embryonic fusion, they can occur following trauma.

C True More commonly they are situated at the base of the nose, forehead, external occipital protuberance and external angle of the eye.

D True They are lined with squamous epithelium and may even contain hair.

E False The congenital variety should always have a preoperative X-ray as they can extend deeply into the cranium and hence dissection under general anaesthetic is required.

113 A True They are associated with excessive exposure to the sun, may progress to frank squamous carcinoma and should be biopsied to exclude malignant transformation.

B True This is an example of carcinoma-in-situ. It can occur anywhere on the body and frequently occurs as a raised, brown, fissured plaque.

C True This is the same pathological entity as Bowen's disease but is confined to the penis and vulva.

D False This is a hereditary condition whereby the individual develops hyperkeratotic palmar and plantar skin, and is associated with the development of oesophageal carcinoma.

E False This condition is not premalignant; however, approximately 10% of these moles develop frank malignant change, hence they should be observed carefully.

(For more information, see ch 17 of Principles and Practice of Surgery)

114 The following skin lesions have an infective origin:
  A senile warts.
  B plantar warts.
  C keratoacanthoma.
  D pyogenic granuloma.
  E leukoplakia.

115 Basal cell carcinoma:
  A metastasises to regional lymph nodes.
  B occurs exclusively on the head and neck.
  C may be clinically confused with a malignant melanoma.
  D histologically is characterised by keratin pearl formation.
  E responds to radiation therapy.

116 Squamous cell carcinoma:
  A metastasises to regional lymph nodes.
  B is commoner than basal cell carcinoma.
  C occurs exclusively on hair-bearing skin.
  D occurs as a late complication in chronic osteomyelitis.
  E commonly occurs in albinos and transplant recipients.

(Answers overleaf)

114 A False   These are greasy, crusty lesions normally situated on the trunk and they have a propensity for crumbling apart and falling off.

B True   These resistant papilloma virus infections are normally contracted from bathing facilities and give rise to pain. They should be treated with curettage or cryotherapy.

C True   These benign self-limiting infective swellings develop at an alarming rate and are frequently mistaken for a squamous carcinoma. They occur most commonly on the face as a hemispherical nodule with a friable red centre.

D True   This is a painful vascular granulation usually present on the fingers or hand and occurs secondary to infection but is not contagious.

E False   This is a premalignant lesion present in the oral mucosa.

115 A False   This neoplasm is locally invasive, only very rarely metastasising to distant sites.

B False   Although the vast majority of lesions occur around the middle third of the face, with a propensity for the inner canthus, they may occur on any hair-bearing skin and the morphoeic or superficial spreading type tends to occur on the trunk.

C True   BCC has a melanotic variant which is easily confused with melanoma; also, melanomas may be amelanotic so the distinction is not always straightforward.

D False   This is the histopathological feature of a squamous cell carcinoma.

E True   BCC responds to external beam radiation although surgery is the mainstay of treatment in most cases.

116 A True   This is the classical mode of spread; however, aggressive neoplasms may metastasise to the liver at an early stage.

B False   BCC occurs three times more commonly.

C False   This neoplasm may occur on any surface normally lined with squamous epithelium, such as the oropharynx, oesophagus, anus and vagina, but also where squamous metaplasia has occurred, e.g. bronchus, bladder.

D True   This is the eponymous Marjolin's ulcer, which will occur following any chronic inflammatory condition, e.g. burn, varicose ulcer, fistula, sinus.

E True   Epidermal carcinoma is the commonest malignancy to occur in transplant recipients. Its behaviour is more aggressive with an earlier age of presentation and it exhibits more metastatic potential.

(For more information, see ch 17 of Principles and Practice of Surgery)

117 Malignant melanoma:
  A when amelanotic behaves more aggressively than usual.
  B may occur on the soles of the feet and palms of the hands.
  C has an incidence of 40 per 100 000 in the Western world.
  D is most commonly of the superficial spreading type.
  E is staged according to its depth of invasion.

118 Malignant melanoma:
  A is more common in females.
  B is extremely rare in dark-skinned races.
  C only arises from the skin.
  D has a worse prognosis when present on the lower limb.
  E for the most part arises de novo on normal skin.

119 Concerning malignant melanoma:
  A stage I disease has a 70% 5-year survival.
  B isolated limb perfusion with chemotherapeutic agents has increased the survival in patients with metastatic disease affecting the lower limb by 25%.
  C the rate of malignant transformation in common moles is 1 per 100 000.
  D >20% of lentigo maligna develop into invasive melanomas.
  E Doppler ultrasound is a useful diagnostic tool.

(Answers overleaf)

117 A True   Amelanotic melanomas are uncommon and include the subungual variant which displays inherently aggressive malignant behaviour with a propensity for early dissemination.

B True   This is the acral variant which constitutes <1% of all melanomas and is common in older individuals and dark-skinned races.

C False   The incidence is presently about 10 per 100 000 and is increasing rapidly in the Western world.

D True   Superficial spreading melanoma constitutes approximately 65% of cases.

E True   Breslow's classification is used ubiquitously in staging the disease locally. In terms of 5-year survival — <1.5 mm (93%), 1.5–3.5 mm (60%), >3.5 mm (48%). When regional nodes or metastases are present survival is 30% and 0% respectively.

118 A True   Approximately 2:1. This is on account of the increasing incidence of lower limb melanomas in young women. Men develop trunk melanomas more commonly.

B True

C False   It occurs in any tissue containing melanocytes, e.g. retina, anus, oesophagus, bronchus.

D False   The disease behaves more aggressively on the trunk, head and neck.

E False   50% arise in junctional naevi.

119 A True

B False   Despite much early enthusiasm over the employment of isolated limb perfusion and the use of strategies such as lymphokine-activated T-cell innoculation, the survival has been improved by only 10% in this patient population.

C True

D False   Approximately 5% of lentigo maligna progress to frank melanoma. Lentigo maligna occurs in older individuals and can be managed expectantly.

E True   Melanomas have an excellent blood supply and when >1 mm in depth will give an excellent signal and will help differentiate benign pigmented naevi from melanomas.

(For more information, see ch 17 of Principles and Practice of Surgery)

120 The following statements are true:

A   cirsoid aneurysm is a self-limiting haemangioma of childhood.

B   von Recklinghausen's disease is inherited as an autosomal recessive condition.

C   hidradenitis suppurativa is a chronic infection of apocrine glands which results in intradermal abscess formation leading to sinus formation.

D   Dupuytren's contracture occurs as a result of thickening of the flexor retinaculum.

E   carpal tunnel syndrome occurs more frequently in females.

(Answers overleaf)

120 A False It is a tortuous venous abnormality fed by an artery occurring commonly on the scalp. It may penetrate the skull and communicate with a similar vascular malformation in the epidural space.

    B False This condition has an autosomal dominant inheritance pattern.

    C True This condition affects the axillae, perineum or groin and may respond to long-term antibiotics, but ultimately may require excision of the skin and grafting.

    D False This results from thickening of the palmer or plantar aponeurosis and occurs in alcoholics, epileptics or as an idiopathic phenomenon.

    E True This condition occurs commonly in pregnancy and in women taking the oral contraceptive pill. It also occurs in acromegaly, hypothyroidism, rheumatoid arthritis and following Colles' fracture.

(For more information, see ch 17 of Principles and Practice of Surgery)

13. The breast

121 Mastalgia:
   A of a cyclical variety is more common in younger women.
   B which is noncyclical is responsive to injection of local anaesthetic and steroid cocktail in over 50% of cases.
   C is the only presenting symptom in 15% of women with breast cancer.
   D of a cyclical nature is associated with an abnormal plasma fatty acid profile.
   E of a cyclical nature normally resolves after parity.

122 The following drugs are useful in the treatment of cyclical mastalgia:
   A danazol.
   B gamolenic acid.
   C diuretics.
   D progestogens.
   E tamoxifen.

(Answers overleaf)

121 **A** **True**   The average age for cyclical breast pain is 34 years compared with noncyclical pain which is 43 years. Cyclical breast pain occurs twice as commonly as noncyclical pain.

B **False**   Noncyclical breast pain can be categorised as: (a) localised to the chest wall; (b) referred pain; (c) true diffuse breast pain. Only pain localised to the chest wall with a specific trigger point will obtain relief from this form of therapy in 60% of cases.

C **False**   It may be seen in inflammatory carcinoma of the breast or when there is skin involvement; however, only 7% of patients with breast cancer have mastalgia as their only symptom.

D **True**   Women with cyclical mastalgia have been shown to have abnormal plasma fatty acid profiles. Gamolenic acid alters the natural fatty acid profile.

E **False**   Cyclical mastalgia is relieved by the menopause, but parity and pregnancy do not affect its course.

122 **A** **True**   100 mg of danazol (Danol) given daily on days 14–28 of the menstrual cycle will produce a response in approximately 80% of patients with cyclical mastalgia. 30% of patients develop side effects — acne, hirsutism and weight gain.

B **True**   Gamolenic acid offers a response rate of 38% in patients with both cyclical and noncyclical mastalgia, with morbidity occurring in only 4% of individuals.

C **False**   Although many women report breast swelling and abdominal bloating in the luteal phase of the menstrual cycle, there is no scientific evidence showing an increase in the total body water between patients with mastalgia and controls.

D **False**   Progestogens have been used both topically and orally and have been shown to be ineffective.

E **True**   Both tamoxifen and goserelin (a gonadotrophin releasing hormone agonist) have been shown to be effective in treating cyclical mastalgia, but neither is currently licensed for treatment of this condition in the UK.

(For more information, see ch 18 of Principles and Practice of Surgery)

123 Breast infection:
  A should be treated by antibiotics in the first instance to abort abscess formation.
  B progressing to abscess formation should be treated by aspiration in the first instance.
  C occurring in neonates is usually caused by *E. coli*.
  D due to periductal mastitis is strongly associated with smoking.
  E in the post-partum period is a contraindication to breast feeding.

124 Fibroadenomata of the breast:
  A of <2 cm will resolve spontaneously in 50% of patients.
  B arise from aberrant development of a lobule.
  C are hypermobile swellings with a peak incidence in the second and third decades.
  D have the potential for malignant transformation.
  E should be confirmed by fine-needle cytology to exclude cystosarcoma phyloides.

(Answers overleaf)

123 A True   There are four guiding principles in treating breast
                   infection: (a) appropriate antibiotics in the first
                   instance to reduce abscess formation; (b) refer to
                   hospital if the infection does not settle rapidly
                   on antibiotics; (c) if abscess is suspected then
                   aspiration should be attempted prior to surgical
                   drainage; (d) inflammatory breast cancer should be
                   excluded.
    B True   This may be repeated.
    C False   *Staph. aureus* is the commonest infecting
                   organism; *E. coli* is an occasional offender, as with
                   other neonatal infections.
    D True   Approximately 90% of women who develop
                   periductal mastitis or its complications smoke,
                   compared with 38% of the same age group in the
                   general population.
    E False   Drainage of milk from the infected segment should
                   be encouraged and is best achieved by continuing
                   breast feeding. An important caveat is that
                   tetracycline, ciprofloxacin and chloramphenicol
                   should be avoided in lactating infection as they can
                   harm the baby.

124 A True   There is evidence that small fibroadenomata will
                   resolve spontaneously, therefore provided the
                   diagnosis has been confirmed cytologically it is
                   reasonable to manage these benign lumps
                   expectantly with 6-monthly review in younger
                   women.
    B True   These are not neoplasms but are the result of
                   abnormal multiplication of ducts and acini.
    C True
    D True   This is extremely rare.
    E True   This is the one situation where the fibroadenoma
                   should be excised. Phyloides tumours have the
                   potential for sarcomatous degeneration and may
                   metastases in 10% of cases.

(For more information, see ch 18 of Principles and Practice of Surgery)

125 Regarding nipple changes in breast disease:
  A split nipples are an acquired phenomenon.
  B breast cancer is the commonest cause of nipple retraction.
  C blood discharging from a single duct is characteristic of an intraduct papilloma.
  D Paget's disease of the nipple is indicative of an underlying intraduct carcinoma.
  E blood discharge should be managed expectantly.

126 Concerning fibrocystic disease of the breast:
  A it is most common in the second decade of life.
  B it is characterised histologically by apocrine metaplasia.
  C carcinoma of the breast is more common in women with this condition.
  D it most commonly affects the upper outer quadrant of the left breast.
  E aspirate from cysts is usually straw-coloured and of use for cytological evaluation.

(Answers overleaf)

125 A False This is mainly congenital.

   B False Mammary duct ectasia is still the commonest cause of nipple retraction. It is important to exclude carcinoma as the first priority when a patient presents with nipple retraction, especially if this is unilateral and the history is short. Mammography is mandatory with careful follow-up.

   C True This is the commonest mode of presentation in intraduct papilloma. Duct ectasia with superimposed infection may also present in this manner, as may an intraduct carcinoma although this is an unusual isolated symptom.

   D True The eczematous periareolar reaction is indicative of Paget's disease and can be confirmed by nipple biopsy where large clear vacuolated cells are present. Paget's disease of the nipple is indicative of an occult intraductal carcinoma or an invasive ductal carcinoma.

   E False Bloody discharge from the nipple should be managed expeditiously.

126 A False It has a peak incidence in late premenopausal and menopausal women.

   B True This is a histological hallmark of fibrocystic disease.

   C True The incidence of carcinoma in the fibrocystic breast is approximately three times that of normal breasts. Atypical hyperplasia is believed to represent the borderline between benign epithelial hyperplasia and carcinoma-in-situ. Malignant transformation has been shown in breasts exhibiting sclerosing adenosis.

   D True This is also the case for carcinoma of the breast.

   E False The content of cysts is classically turbid (green or brown). Cytological assessment is of little value as the smears are usually of poor quality and raise unnecessary confusion over the nature of the swelling.

(For more information, see ch 18 of Principles and Practice of Surgery)

127 The following are true regarding carcinoma of the female breast:

  A it is the second commonest female malignancy.

  B there is a strong geographical variation in disease incidence.

  C 10% of breast cancer in the Western world has a genetic predisposition.

  D long-term use of the oral contraceptive pill increases the risk of premenopausal breast cancer.

  E tamoxifen, taken prophylactically, reduces the risk of breast cancer development.

128 Mammography:

  A is the most sensitive screening tool currently available for detection of breast carcinoma.

  B as a screening tool has been shown to reduce the mortality from breast cancer by 30% in women >50 years.

  C should be exclusively employed in women >50 years.

  D when combined with ultrasonography increases the diagnostic sensitivity of breast lumps.

  E used in screening detects important abnormalities of which over 50% are impalpable.

(Answers overleaf)

127 **A** **False**　This is the commonest female malignancy in economically developed countries and at least 7% of women in the UK will develop breast cancer. It comprises 18% of all female cancers.

B **True**　The age-adjusted incidence and mortality for breast cancer varies by a factor of at least 7 between countries. The incidence is lowest in Japanese women.

C **True**　Breast cancer susceptibility is generally inherited in an autosomal dominant fashion with limited penetrance. About one-third of the familial cases are thought to be due to a mutation in the BRCA1 gene on the long arm of chromosome 17.

D **True**　Young women using the pill for 4 years before their first term pregnancy almost certainly increase the risk of premenopausal breast cancer.

E **True**　It was noticed incidently that tamoxifen reduced the incidence of breast cancer in the contralateral breast in women with breast cancer. Studies comparing tamoxifen with a placebo in women at high risk of breast cancer are currently underway.

128 **A** **True**　There is no evidence that clinical examination, ultrasonography and teaching self examination of the breast are effective tools in screening for breast cancer. A UK national programme now offers mammography every 3 years to women aged 50–64.

B **True**　Combined trials in Sweden have shown an overall reduction in breast cancer mortality of 29% during 12 years of follow-up in women >50 years and a 13% reduction in younger women.

C **False**　High risk individuals who are younger should also be offered screening, despite the difficulty with interpretation of mammography.

D **True**　Ultrasonography has the added advantage of being able to detect cystic lesions which are generally benign.

E **True**　70% of lesions diagnosed by mammography are impalpable. This necessitates the use of image guided fine-needle aspiration or stereotactic biopsy.

(For more information, see ch 18 of Principles and Practice of Surgery)

129 A T4b N2 M1 breast cancer will have the following features:
- **A** tumour mass >5 cm.
- **B** a contralateral neoplasm.
- **C** involved lymph nodes in the contralateral axilla.
- **D** distant metastases.
- **E** skin involvement on the ipsilateral side.

130 In breast cancer:
- **A** histological features of nuclear pleomorphism and frequent mitotic figures are bad prognostic indicators.
- **B** medullary carcinoma has a grave prognosis.
- **C** level III axillary clearance provides a lower rate of axillary recurrence than radiotherapy to the axilla.
- **D** radiotherapy decreases the risk of locoregional recurrence.
- **E** axillary staging is mandatory for all premenopausal patients.

(Answers overleaf)

129 **A False**   A T3 tumour is >5 cm. T4 infers a tumour of any
size which extends directly to the chest wall or skin.

    B False

    C False   N2 implies fixed ipsilateral lymph nodes.

    D True   M1 implies distant metastases or dissemination to
supraclavicular lymph nodes.

    E True   4b implies either peau d'orange or the presence of
satellite skin nodules in the same breast.

130 **A True**   These parameters, plus attempts at tubule
formation, are histopathological criteria used in the
Nottingham index for grading breast cancers.

    B False   Lobular, tubular, cribriform and medullary
carcinoma are all associated with a better prognosis. Medullary carcinoma constitutes approximately 7% of all breast carcinomas.

    C True   Axillary clearance affords excellent control of
disease. In a 10-year period there is a 3% recurrence
after axillary clearance, 8% recurrence after
radiotherapy alone and 21% recurrence when the
management has been purely expectant.

    D True   It has been shown to reduce the incidence of locally
recurrent disease by approximately 40%.

    E True   This is crucial to the staging process and is an
important criterion when considering adjuvant
chemotherapy.

(For more information, see ch 18 of Principles and Practice of Surgery)

14. Endocrine surgery

131 Concerning thyroid enlargement:
- **A** transient enlargement may occur during pregnancy.
- **B** the aetiology may be infective in origin.
- **C** multinodular goitre is frequently associated with myxoedema.
- **D** goitre of Graves' disease frequently causes pressure symptoms.
- **E** malignant transformation occurs in 5% of multinodular goitres.

132 Hashimoto's disease:
- **A** has a strong female preponderance.
- **B** has its diagnosis confirmed by the presence of high plasma titres of anti-smooth muscle antibodies.
- **C** may be associated with the presence of skin hypo-pigmentation.
- **D** predisposes the patient to the late development of anaplastic carcinoma.
- **E** frequently results in hypothyroidism.

133 In solitary thyroid nodules:
- **A** 10% of hot (functioning) nodules are malignant.
- **B** Fine-needle cytology is sensitive in diagnosing follicular carcinomas.
- **C** preoperative X-rays of the thoracic inlet are mandatory.
- **D** there is a 10% chance of malignancy in all age groups.
- **E** radioisotope scan is the most important preoperative investigation.

(Answers overleaf)

131 A True   Increased demands for thyroxine, increased renal
clearance of iodine and changes in serum proteins
contribute to this physiological goitre.

B True   This is seen in De Quervain's thyroiditis which is
due to a viral infection. It results in a diffuse painful
swelling of the gland and runs a fluctuating
although self-limiting course.

C False   Quite the converse; multinodular goitre is more
commonly associated with hyperthyroidism.

D False   The enlargement seen in Graves' disease results in
a small hypervascular goitre.

E True

132 A True   Postmenopausal females are usually affected
(female-to-male ratio 10:1).

B False   The diagnosis depends on the demonstration of
high titres of antibodies to microsomal components
of follicular cells. Antibodies to thyroglobulin and
thyroid cell cytosol are also detectable in the serum.

C True   As with any autoimmune disease, vitiligo may
occur.

D False   Lymphoma may develop in long-standing
Hashimoto's disease.

E True   In the initial stages of the disease the patient may
be slightly thyrotoxic; however, as the disease
'burns out' the patient develops hypothyroidism.

133 A False   10% of cold (nonfunctioning) nodules are
malignant; however, only 1% of hot nodules are
malignant. In true solitary nodules, 50%
are cysts and the rest are adenomata or
differentiated malignancies.

B False   Fine-needle aspiration is of limited value in
differentiating between follicular adenoma and
carcinoma. One must assess the capsule of the
nodule histologically to confirm or exclude capsular
invasion.

C False   Thoracic inlet views are only indicated if the patient
has stridor, dysphagia, hoarseness or evidence of
plunging retrosternal extension.

D False   Solitary thyroid nodules have a female preponderance (4:1) and commonly present between 30
and 50 years. Approximately 10% of these nodules
are malignant in this age group, but the figure
exceeds 50% in the extremes of life.

E False   Although this was once considered to be useful it
will not influence the decision to operate as even
hot nodules have a low incidence of malignancy.

(For more information, see ch 19 of Principles and Practice of Surgery)

134 In thyrotoxicosis:
  A Lugol's iodine inhibits thyroid hormone release and can be employed in long-term treatment.
  B due to Graves' disease, the TSH receptor on the surface follicular cells is the prime autoantigen.
  C free thryroxine levels may be within normal limits.
  D ophthalmopathy occurs in 10% of patients with Graves' disease.
  E β-blockers have no specific effects on thyroxine metabolism but are useful indirectly in controlling symptoms.

135 The following are true of malignant tumours of the thyroid gland:
  A papillary carcinoma is best managed by hemithyroidectomy and adjuvant I^{131}.
  B follicular carcinoma has a propensity for blood-borne spread and hence a worse prognosis than papillary carcinoma.
  C medullary carcinoma may exhibit an autosomal recessive inheritance pattern.
  D anaplastic carcinoma tends to occur in the elderly population and has a propensity for early local invasion.
  E papillary and medullary carcinoma have a propensity for lymph node dissemination.

136 Primary hyperparathyroidism:
  A results in dystrophic calcification.
  B causes tetany.
  C has the following serum bone profile: calcium increased, phosphate increased, alkaline phosphatase decreased.
  D is the result of parathyroid hyperplasia in 90% of cases.
  E may result in brown tumour formation.

(Answers overleaf)

134 **A** **False**   The effects of Lugol's iodine are short-lived, lasting 2 weeks; however, it is employed for 10–14 days to reduce the vascularity of the gland, preoperatively.

B **True**

C **True**   In T3 thyrotoxicosis thyroxine levels will be within normal limits. Tri-iodothyronine will be elevated and TSH suppressed.

D **False**   Ophthalmic signs occur in approximately 30% of patients. This may result in exophthalmos, proptosis, strabismus, diplopia, papilloedema, retinal haemorrhage, exposure keratitis and consequently decreased visual acuity.

E **False**   β-adrenergic blocking agents interfere with the peripheral conversion of T4 to T3. They also control many of the manifestations of hyperthyroidism.

135 **A** **False**   Papillary carcinoma may be multifocal, and despite a palpably normal contralateral lobe at operation there is still a chance of residual disease thus total thyroidectomy should be performed.

B **True**

C **False**   MEN IIa syndrome has an autosomal dominant inheritance pattern (Sipples syndrome) and comprises medullary carcinoma, phaeo-chromocytoma and parathyroid adenomas.

D **True**   It frequently involves the recurrent laryngeal nerve, compresses the oesophagus and trachea and may occasionally invade the cervical sympathetic chain causing Horner's syndrome.

E **True**

136 **A** **False**   This refers to calcium deposition in dead tissue; calcium metabolism is normal, however.

B **False**   Tetany is a feature of hypocalcaemia.

C **False**   Parathormone is phosphaturic, hence phosphate excretion in the urine is increased and the plasma level is reduced. Alkaline phosphatase is increased as bone resorption is increased.

D **False**   It is due to a parathyroid adenoma in 90% of cases, 20% of which are multiple; parathyroid hyperplasia accounts for approximately 9%, and parathyroid carcinoma <1%.

E **True**   This is part of the condition von Recklinghausen's disease of bone (osteitis cystica generalisata) where bone resorption occurs in the mandible (brown tumour).

(For more information, see ch 19 of Principles and Practice of Surgery)

137 Hypercalcaemia:

A occurs in secondary hyperparathyroidism.
B may occur as an early complication of total thyroidectomy.
C occurs in acute haemorrhagic pancreatitis.
D due to primary hyperparathyroidism responds to steroid therapy.
E occurs in sarcoidosis.

138 Cushing's syndrome:

A is more commonly due to primary malfunction of the pituitary gland than of the adrenal glands.
B results in hypokalaemia.
C due to a pituitary adenoma will repond to the high dexamethasone suppression test.
D when treated inappropriately by bilateral adrenalectomy will result in skin hyperpigmentation.
E may occur in association with bronchogenic carcinoma.

(Answers overleaf)

137 A False   In secondary hyperparathyroidism there is hypersecretion of parathormone in response to low circulating levels of ionised calcium. This is usually the result of renal disease or malabsorption.
    B False   Transient hypocalcaemia may occur.
    C False   Hypercalcaemia is a predisposing factor for pancreatitis. In pancreatitis, hypocalcaemia may occur.
    D False   If hypercalcaemia improves with systemic steroids then the diagnosis is not primary hyper-parathryoidism. Hypercalcaemia of malignancy responds dramatically to steroid therapy.
    E True

138 A True   Pituitary adenoma (79%), adrenal adenoma (19%), adrenal carcinoma (1%), ectopic ACTH secretion (1%) and finally primary adrenal hyperplasia all cause Cushing's syndrome.
    B True   Due to the mineralocorticoid effect, sodium is retained at the expense of potassium secretion in the renal tubules.
    C False   Dexamethasone (2 mg q.i.d. for 48 hours) will suppress the production of ACTH from a pituitary adenoma, resulting in a decrease in urinary and plasma cortisols, but it will have no effect on the secretion from a primary adrenal tumour or from an ectopic source.
    D True   This is Nelson's syndrome. If the end organ is removed then positive feedback results in increased secretion of ACTH from the adenoma in the anterior pituitary, producing abnormal skin pigmentation.
    E True   This is ectopic ACTH secretion which can occur as a paraneoplastic phenomenon seen with several tumours (e.g. pancreas, thymus).

(For more information, see ch 19 of Principles and Practice of Surgery)

139 Phaeochromocytoma:
   A arises from the chromaffin cells of the adrenal medulla.
   B is always benign.
   C is exclusive to the adrenal medulla.
   D is a recognised cause of sudden death.
   E may be diagnosed by nuclear scintigraphy using
         radiolabelled iodine.

140 The following statements are true:
   A Addison's disease may occur secondary to bronchogenic
         carcinoma.
   B hypotension is a feature of Conn's disease.
   C neuroblastoma is the commonest solid childhood
         malignancy.
   D secondary disease from a carcinoid tumour is necessary
         before the systemic effects of the carcinoid syndrome can
         occur.
   E there is no place for hepatic resection in the treatment of
         the carcinoid syndrome.

(Answers overleaf)

139 **A True**

    B False   10% of tumours are malignant, 10% are familial, 10% are multiple and 10% arise outside the adrenal gland in the sympathetic chain.

    C False

    D True   Sudden hypertensive crises may result in sudden death. This is well recognised in pregnancy and in the perioperative period, especially if the condition is occult.

    E True   Ultrasonography, CT scanning, selective venous sampling, urinary assay for 3-methoxy-4-mandelic acid (VMA) and, more recently, meta-iodobenzyl-guanidine (MIBG) scanning are employed in the diagnosis of phaeochromocytoma.

140 **A True**   The adrenals are a common site for secondary spread from carcinoma of the bronchus and breast.

    B False   Conn's disease occurs as a result of an adrenal cortex adenoma which secretes aldosterone. Hypertension occurs due to the mineralocorticoid effect.

    C True   This is an aggressive neoplasm occurring in primitive cells of the adrenal gland and sympathetic chain. It spreads both to lymphatics and haematogenously to lungs and bone (40%).

    D False   5-hydroxy-tryptamine is cleared by 'first pass' in the liver. Primary carcinoid tumours also arise in the bronchus and hence the syndrome of flushing, bronchospasm and diarrhoea can occur without secondary deposition.

    E False   The mainstay of treatment of the carcinoid syndrome is to control the symptoms. Medical therapy with somatostatin, hepatic resection, hepatic artery embolisation and, more recently, orthotopic liver transplantation are all successfully employed.

(For more information, see ch 19 of Principles and Practice of Surgery)

15. Cardiac surgery

Peripheral vascular disease

141 Coronary artery bypass grafting:
- **A** is associated with an operative mortality rate of 5–8% in patients under 70 years.
- **B** produces complete relief from angina symptoms in over 90% of patients.
- **C** is associated with relief from angina which is usually permanent.
- **D** involves insertion of prosthetic grafts between the aorta and coronary arteries.
- **E** usually involves the use of cardiopulmonary bypass and cardioplegic arrest of the heart.

142 Complications of coronary artery occlusion include:
- **A** myocardial infarction.
- **B** cardiogenic shock.
- **C** ventricular aneurysm.
- **D** muscle rupture.
- **E** conduction defects.

143 Concerning congenital heart disease:
- **A** it occurs in less than 1 per 1000 live births.
- **B** coarctation of the aorta usually occurs proximal to the origin of the left subclavian artery.
- **C** ventricular septal defects cause right-to-left shunting of blood.
- **D** a patent ductus arteriosus may cause cardiac failure in infancy.
- **E** tetralogy of Fallot results in right-to-left shunting and cyanosis.

(Answers overleaf)

141 **A** **False** The operative mortality rate is 1–2%.
     B **False** Complete relief from angina is obtained in 60–80% of patients.
     C **False** Angina gradually returns, so that only 30–50% are symptom-free at 10 years.
     D **False** The saphenous vein may be used, but the internal mammary arteries are preferred as their use is associated with a lower incidence of graft occlusion.
     E **True**

142 **A** **True**
     B **True** Due to infarction of left ventricular muscle.
     C **True** This is a late complication due to replacement of ventricular muscle by a weak fibrous scar.
     D **True** This may result in an interventricular septal defect if this is the area of muscle involved, or mitral regurgitation if a papillary muscle is involved.
     E **True**

143 **A** **False** It occurs in approximately 6–8 per 1000 live births.
     B **False** It usually occurs just beyond it.
     C **False** Shunting occurs in the opposite direction because pressure in the left ventricle is higher than in the right during systole.
     D **True** Due to left-to-right shunting of systemic blood into the pulmonary circulation.
     E **True** Due to malalignment of the aorta and pulmonary artery over the interventricular septum.

(For more information, see chs 20 and 21 of Principles and Practice of Surgery)

144 Concerning valvular heart disease:

A mitral valve disease is usually due to infarction and rupture of a papillary muscle.

B aortic valve disease may occur following syphilis and a dissecting aortic aneurysm.

C pulmonary valve disease is usually due to rheumatic fever.

D following insertion of prosthetic mechanical valves, indefinite oral anticoagulation is required.

E prosthetic valves are associated with a risk of infective endocarditis.

145 Concerning nonoperative treatment of obliterative disease of the lower limbs:

A antiplatelet therapy may be beneficial.

B vasodilatory drugs may be beneficial.

C sympathectomy may increase muscle blood flow and improve claudication pain.

D percutaneous angioplasty is applicable for dilating a long structure.

E naftidrofuryl oxalate (Praxilene) may improve claudication.

146 Surgical treatment of obliterative arterial disease of the lower limb may involve:

A thromboendarterectomy.

B aorto-femoral vein graft to bypass an iliac lesion.

C femoro-femoral crossover graft to bypass an iliac lesion.

D femoro-popliteal bypass using the saphenous vein.

E amputation.

(Answers overleaf)

144 **A False**   It is usually due to rheumatic fever.
  B True   These may be associated with aortic incompetence.
  C False   It is usually a congenital stenosis.
  D True   Warfarin is used. Porcine xenografts do not require prophylatic anticogulation.
  E True   Prophylactic antibiotics should be administered at times of potential bacteraemia, e.g. dental manipulation or urinary instrumentation.

145 **A True**   For example, aspirin, 300 mg per day.
  B False   These are of no benefit.
  C False   This may improve skin blood flow thus possibly relieving coldness and rest pain. It does not increase muscle blood flow.
  D False   It is only applicable for short stenoses.
  E True   It may be worth a trial in elderly patients with claudication for whom no other active intervention is possible.

146 **A True**   To remove local atherosclerotic plaque and thrombus.
  B False   This is the appropriate anatomical bypass, but a prosthetic graft (e.g. Dacron) is used.
  C True   This is an example of an 'extra-anatomic' bypass, i.e. it does not follow the normal anatomical path. This may be used when an iliac artery is blocked and the patient is unfit for abdominal surgery such as an aorto-femoral Dacron graft.
  D True   For example, to bypass a lesion in the superficial femoral artery. Prosthetic grafts (e.g. PTFE) may also be used, but the saphenous vein is associated with a lower graft thrombosis rate.
  E True   If arterial reconstruction for limb salvage has failed or is not possible.

(For more information, see chs 20 and 21 of Principles and Practice of Surgery)

147 Acute arterial occlusion:

A   may be caused by thrombosis or embolism.
B   when due to embolus, is usually associated with atrial fibrillation.
C   usually presents initially with paraesthesia and loss of power in the limb.
D   should be treated by emergency thrombectomy/ embolectomy if there are signs of severe ischaemia.
E   may be treated with thrombolytic therapy given systemically.

148 Concerning aneurysms:

A   a true aneurysm is covered by all three layers of the vessel wall.
B   a dissecting aneurysm occurs due to destruction of the vessel intima.
C   an aortic aneurysm usually occurs above the level of the renal arteries.
D   an aortic aneurysm >6 cm diameter should be repaired.
E   pain due to aortic aneurysm rupture may mimic renal colic.

149 Varicose veins:

A   occur more frequently in men than in women.
B   may be associated with chronic skin changes.
C   in the thigh may be treated by injection sclerotherapy.
D   may be associated with chronic leg ulceration, typically on the lateral aspect of the leg.
E   may be tested clinically using the Trendelenberg test to detect the level of superficial-to-deep reflux through incompetent perforators.

(Answers overleaf)

147 A True   Trauma or dissecting aneurysm may also be responsible.

B True   It may also be associated with cardiac failure or recent myocardial infarction.

C False   Coldness and pain are usually the first symptoms, followed by paraesthesia, loss of sensation and loss of power.

D True   These include loss of power, loss of sensation and muscle tenderness.

E False   Thrombolytic therapy (e.g. streptokinase, urokinase or tissue plasminogen activator) is given directly into the artery and thrombus by percutaneous catheter, under radiological control.

148 A True   A false aneurysm occurs when an artery is pierced resulting in a surrounding haematoma which remains in continuity with the vessel lumen.

B False   Destruction of the media results in dissection with blood in this plane.

C False   95% are below this level.

D True   Provided the patient is fit — using a prosthetic graft.

E True   Hence a high index of suspicion is necessary, particularly with elderly, hypertensive patients where urinalysis is negative.

149 A False   The female-to-male ratio is 5:1.

B True   These are due to sustained high pressure in the superficial veins and are known as lipodermatosclerosis; this consists of oedema, inflammation, fibrosis, pigmentation and ulceration, depending on the severity.

C False   Sclerotherapy is used for varicosities below the knee. If used for those above the knee, associated with saphenofemoral incompetence, recurrence is inevitable.

D False   Chronic leg ulceration represents the end stage of lipodermatosclerosis but typically occurs on the medial aspect.

E False   The Trendelenberg test detects deep-to-superficial reflux.

(For more information, see chs 20 and 21 of Principles and Practice of Surgery)

150 Venous thrombosis of the lower limb:

   A always involves the deep venous system.
   B is rare in modern surgical practice with the use of heparin
         prophylaxis.
   C occurs more frequently in patients with malignant disease.
   D is most accurately diagnosed by detailed clinical
         examination, including Homan's test.
   E should be treated at an early stage by anticoagulation with
         warfarin.

(Answers overleaf)

150 A False It may consist of a superficial thrombophlebitis —
treatment consists of analgesics, support stockings,
NSAIDs and active exercises.

B False DVT remains a common complication after major
surgery — it may occur in up to 30% of patients
undergoing prolonged intra-abdominal procedures.

C True Due to hypercoagulability of the blood; the other
major aetiological factors are venous stasis and
intimal damage (Virchow's triad).

D False Accurate diagnosis requires venography, which is
performed by injecting contrast into a vein on
the dorsum of the foot, with a tourniquet above the
ankle to direct contrast into the deep system. The
radiofibrinogen uptake test is extremely accurate
but its use is confined to research studies.

E False Heparin is used in the first 5–7 days, after which
the patient is treated with warfarin.

(For more information, see chs 20 and 21 of Principles and Practice of Surgery)

16. The chest and mediastinum

151 Basic airway management may involve the following techniques:

   A chin lift, which involves grasping the angles of the mandible, one hand on each side, and displacing the mandible forwards.

   B hyperextension of the neck to assist the chin lift manoeuvre.

   C suction.

   D an oropharyngeal (Guedel) airway in a patient with a normal gag reflex.

   E a nasopharyngeal airway in a patient with a normal gag reflex.

152 Pneumothorax:

   A may occur spontaneously.

   B should always be treated by intercostal tube drainage.

   C may progress to a tension pneumothorax if there is a large open wound on the chest wall communicating with the exterior.

   D can only occur if air enters the pleural space from the lung or from the exterior.

   E when due to trauma, occurs only with penetrating trauma.

153 Empyema of the chest:

   A refers to a large collection of pus within one or more lobes of the lung.

   B is most commonly due to infection introduced via chest drains.

   C may arise secondary to infection in the mediastinum.

   D should be treated primarily by aggressive antibiotic therapy.

   E may lead ultimately to fibrosis around the lung, with restriction of expansion.

(Answers overleaf)

151 A False This describes the *jaw thrust*. The chin lift involves placing the fingers of one hand under the mandible while the thumb of the same hand depresses the lower lip and incisors to open the mouth.

B False Hyperextension of the neck should not be performed, particularly in a trauma patient with a risk of cervical spine injury.

C True A rigid sucker (and finger, if necessary) should be used to clear blood, secretions, vomitus and foreign bodies from the airway.

D False A patient with a normal gag reflex will not tolerate an oropharyngeal airway.

E True If a Guedel airway is not tolerated a nasopharyngeal airway may be used.

152 A True Particularly in tall, thin patients — if this becomes a recurrent problem the patient may require a pleurodesis or pleurectomy.

B False If there is only a small amount of air in the pleural space, aspiration (needle thoracocentesis) may be sufficient.

C False This results in a sucking chest wound. A tension pneumothorax occurs when the site of air leak in the lung acts as a flap valve allowing air to enter the pleural space, but preventing it from escape during expiration

D False Air could enter the pleural space from a ruptured oesophagus.

E False It may occur with blunt trauma, in association with rib fractures or lung contusion.

153 A False This is a lung abscess. Empyema refers to the presence of pus in the pleural cavity.

B False The commonest cause is pneumonia, with spread of infection into an associated pleural effusion.

C True For example, secondary to a perforated oesophagus.

D False As with any collection of pus, primary treatment involves surgical drainage.

E True Due to organisation and thickening of granulation tissue lining the empyema. Thoracotomy and excision of this may be necessary ('decortication').

(For more information, see ch 22 of Principles and Practice of Surgery)

154 Concerning infective lung conditions:

A empyema and bronchiectasis may be associated with finger clubbing.

B lung abscess may produce a classical appearance on chest X-ray.

C abscess may occur within an area of pneumonia.

D bronchiectasis most commonly affects the upper lobes.

E bronchiectasis is generally treated by postural drainage and antibiotics.

155 Lung cancer:

A affects men more frequently than women with a ratio of 2:1.

B has cigarette smoking as its major predisposing factor in virtually all cases.

C often spreads early by the lymphatics.

D is most frequently an adenocarcinoma.

E often spreads via the blood to the brain and bone.

156 Lung cancer:

A may be associated with peripheral neuropathy.

B may be associated with a cushingoid appearance.

C may be associated with superficial thrombophlebitis.

D may be associated with Horner's syndrome if the lesion is close to the hilum.

E may produce hoarseness usually due to involvement of the right recurrent laryngeal nerve.

157 Lung cancer:

A may be associated with venous engorgement of the face, arms and anterior chest wall.

B often requires bronchoscopy for confirmation of the diagnosis.

C is generally treated by surgical resection, if possible.

D is often treated by chemotherapy.

E when treated by surgical resection is associated with a 5-year survival rate of approximately 80%.

(Answers overleaf)

154 **A** **True**
  B **True**   An opacity containing an air/fluid level.
  C **True**   Although with antibiotic treatment and aggressive physiotherapy for pneumonia, this is rare.
  D **False**   The lower lobes are most commonly affected but it may be widespread.
  E **True**   This is the mainstay of treatment. Occasionally, surgical resection of an affected lobe or segment may be very successful if the disease is localised.

155 **A** **False**   The ratio is 4:1.
  B **True**   A few are also related to asbestos, arsenic or radioactive isotope exposure.
  C **True**   To the hilar and mediastinal lymph nodes and later to the supraclavicular lymph nodes.
  D **False**   The most frequent type is squamous carcinoma (45%), followed by anaplastic carcinoma (35%) and adenocarcinoma (20%). The anaplastic type is further subdivided into large cell (15%) and small or oat cell (20%).
  E **True**   The common sites for blood-borne metastases are brain, bone, liver, skin and the adrenal glands.

156 **A** **True**   All of **A–C** represent systemic manifestations
  B **True**   of lung cancer not due to metastatic disease.
  C **True**   Others include hypertrophic pulmonary osteodystrophy, finger clubbing and endocrine disturbances (e.g. Cushing's syndrome and excess ADH secretion) due to inappropriate secretion of hormones.
  D **False**   This occurs with an apical lesion (Pancoast syndrome) — it is sometimes associated with arm pain due to involvement of the brachial plexus.
  E **False**   It is usually due to involvement of the left recurrent laryngeal nerve.

157 **A** **True**   Due to occlusion of the superior vena cava.
  B **True**   This is suitable for centrally situated lesions. Percutaneous needle biopsy or thoracoscopy is usually required for peripherally situated lesions.
  C **True**   This offers the only hope of cure.
  D **False**   Only small cell tumours are responsive to chemotherapy. The other types are not responsive.
  E **False**   It is only 35–40%.

(For more information, see ch 22 of Principles and Practice of Surgery)

158 Concerning thoracic trauma:

  A approximately 85% of patients with a haemothorax require a thoracotomy.

  B fracture of three or more ribs results in a flail chest.

  C rib fracture alone is not associated with significant morbidity or mortality.

  D aortic rupture should be suspected if there is widening of the upper mediastinum on a chest X-ray.

  E haemothorax should be treated by insertion of an intercostal drain in the 3rd intercostal space, mid-clavicular line.

159 A mass in the mediastinum:

  A if situated in the posterior aspect may be due to a goitre.

  B is usually due to benign disease.

  C if situated in the posterior mediastinum may arise from within the abdomen.

  D if situated in the posterior mediastinum may be biopsied by mediastinoscopy.

  E due to a neurogenic tumour, is usually found in the anterior aspect.

160 On a chest X-ray:

  A a tension pneumothorax will produce deviation of the mediastinum and trachea towards that side.

  B elevation of a hemidiaphragm may occur in patients with hilar carcinoma.

  C a 'coin lesion' or shadow in a smoker should be presumed to be a bronchial carcinoma until proved otherwise.

  D a diagnosis of bronchiectasis can usually be confirmed.

  E an air/fluid level behind the heart shadow is suggestive of a hiatus hernia.

(Answers overleaf)

158 **A** **False** In the majority of cases intercostal tube drainage alone is required. Thoracotomy is necessary in less than 15% of patients.
      B **False** Flail chest results when a number of adjacent ribs are fractured in more than one place.
      C **False** In elderly patients, rib fracture can be associated with significant morbidity (atelectasis, collapse, infection) and subsequent mortality due to inhibition of chest movement by pain.
      D **True**
      E **False** It should be inserted in the 5th or 6th intercostal space, mid-axillary line.

159 **A** **False** A goitre extends from the neck, retrosternally, into the anterosuperior mediastinum.
      B **False** Mediastinal masses are usually due to malignant disease, either 'primary' (arising in the lymphoid system) or 'secondary' (usually from bronchial carcinoma).
      C **True** For example, a rolling (paraoesophageal) hiatus hernia.
      D **False** This is true for anterior mediastinal masses (e.g. lymph nodes around the carina), but posterior masses require formal thoracotomy.
      E **False** Neurogenic tumours (e.g. neurofibromas) are usually found posteriorly.

160 **A** **False** Deviation will occur to the opposite side.
      B **True** Due to phrenic nerve paralysis.
      C **True**
      D **False** This requires bronchography.
      E **True**

(For more information, see ch 22 of Principles and Practice of Surgery)

17. Head, neck and salivary glands

161 Regarding topographical anatomy of the neck:

A the submental triangle has the mandibular ramus and the digastric muscle as its boundaries.

B the internal jugular vein is the immediate relation of the deep cervical lymph node chain.

C the posterior triangle of the neck has the clavicle as its inferior boundary.

D the facial nerve passes through the stylomastoid foramen before giving a branch to the lacrimal gland.

E the thyroid gland obtains its blood supply entirely from branches of the external carotid artery.

162 Concerning cancers of the head and neck:

A 90% are squamous cell carcinomas.

B approximately 50% of patients with carcinoma of the tongue have lymph node metastases at presentation.

C surgery and radiotherapy are the principal treatment modalities.

D radical neck dissection involves excision of all the lymph nodes in the posterior triangle of the neck.

E the size of the lesion, the extent of the surgery and the consequent defect are the major limiting factors in surgery for malignancies in this region.

(Answers overleaf)

161 **A False**   These are the boundaries of the submandibular triangle.

     B True   Jugulodigastric and jugulo-omohyoid are named nodes within this chain.

     C True   The posterior margin is the lateral border of the trapezius muscle, and the anterior margin the posterior border of the sternocleidomastoid muscle.

     D False   The facial nerve exits the cranium via the internal auditory meatus, traverses the middle ear and gives a branch to the stapedius muscle, chorda tympani and parasympathetic efferent fibres to the ciliary ganglion and lacrimal gland before passing through the stylomastoid foramen.

     E False   The inferior thyroid artery is the first branch of the subclavian artery. In 3% of cases there is a branch from the innominate artery to the inferior aspect of the isthmus, called the thyroidea ima artery.

162 **A True**   Cancers of the head and neck comprise approximately 10% of all human malignancies. 90% are squamous cell carcinomas (skin, larynx, oral cavity, oropharynx and hypopharynx).

     B True   Squamous cell carcinomas have a propensity for early lymph node metastases. The incidence of nodal disease increases with increasing size of the primary tumour.

     C True   Surgery is the gold standard treatment for tumours in this region. Whether planned postoperative radiotherapy is administered will depend on factors such as size and site of the primary tumour, tumour clearance, extracapsular rupture or nodal disease, and involvement of more than one level of cervical nodes.

     D False   Radical neck dissection involves the removal of nodes from both the anterior and posterior triangles of the neck, along with the sternomastoid muscle, internal jugular vein and spinal accessory nerve.

     E False   Split-skin grafts, axial skin flaps, e.g. myo-cutaneous flaps, and more recently free micro-vascular transfer of tissue have revolutionised surgery of this region.

(For more information, see ch 23 of Principles and Practice of Surgery)

163   The following are true of fine-needle aspiration (FNA) cytology:
  A as a diagnostic tool in head and neck swellings it is preferred to surgical biopsy.
  B it is quick, accurate, inexpensive and can be carried out in outpatients.
  C it has surpassed lymph node biopsy as the diagnostic method of choice in typing malignant lymphoma.
  D it is especially accurate in cystic neck swellings.
  E tight cellular cohesion of the cellular aspirate is characteristic of malignant swellings.

164   Thyroglossal cysts:
  A are persistent remnants of the tract along which the thyroid gland descends during its embryological development.
  B are exclusive to the midline in the anterior triangle of the neck.
  C move up on protrusion of the tongue.
  D are prone to infection.
  E should be aspirated or incised and drained.

165   The following are differential diagnoses of a midline swelling of the neck:
  A dermoid cyst.
  B submental lymph node.
  C branchial cyst.
  D cystic hygroma.
  E laryngocoele.

(Answers overleaf)

163 A True   Surgical biopsy is often contraindicated in the head and neck region because of the risks of facial nerve damage, fistula formation or tumour seeding.

B True   The main attraction is that the patient can have a diagnosis expeditiously.

C False   Although FNA can be used to differentiate between lymphoma, secondary carcinoma and inflammatory disease it cannot type lymphomas specifically.

D False   FNA has low sensitivity in cystic swellings. Metastatic squamous cell carcinomas, metastatic papillary thyroid carcinomas and salivary gland tumours may all have a cystic component.

E False   Benign epithelium exhibits contact inhibition and is usually present in sheets. One of the first biological features of malignant transformation is loss of contact inhibition, hence cells tend to separate easily.

164 A True   The thyroglossal tract should atrophy completely; however, any persistence will form a cyst or develop into ectopic thyroid tissue in the middle of the neck.

B False   Although the classical site is in the midline, the cyst may be displaced to either side by the thyroid cartilage.

C True   Because of the attachment to the hyoid bone.

D True   These cysts are lined with ciliated respiratory epithelium and are prone to infection.

E False   Simple drainage or incomplete excision will result in a persistent discharging sinus. Incision and drainage is reserved for frank abscess formation. Excision is recommended.

165 A True   These are usually lower in the neck and have no deep attachment.

B True   These are frequently situated in the midline.

C False   These occur laterally on the anterior border of the upper third of the sternomastoid.

D False   This is the classical neck mass at birth. This lymphangiomatous tissue also extends into the axilla, and the pectoral, buccal and parotid regions.

E False   This is a lateral swelling of the larynx seen in trumpet and other wind instrument players. It is usually bilateral and of little clinical significance.

(For more information, see ch 23 of Principles and Practice of Surgery)

166 Branchial cysts:

   A are derived from ectoderm of the second branchial pouch.

   B are situated at the posterior border of the lower third of the sternocleidomastoid muscle.

   C are lined with squamous epithelium and contain cholesterol crystals.

   D may have an external opening at the anterior border of the lower third of the sternocleidomastoid.

   E may have an associated tract which extends deeply between the internal and external carotid arteries.

167 The following are true of salivary neoplasms:

   A they have an incidence of 4 per 100 000.

   B tumours of the minor salivary glands are more likely to be benign than tumours arising in the major salivary glands.

   C adenolymphoma (Warthin's tumour) is a malignant condition.

   D adenoid cystic carcinoma classically presents as a painless swelling of the parotid gland.

   E pleomorphic adenomas have potential for malignant transformation.

168 The following are true of parotid neoplasms:

   A pleomorphic adenomas constitute over 60% of tumours at this site.

   B pleomorphic adenomas are well encapsulated, hence are best treated by local excision.

   C adenoid cystic carcinomas are the commonest malignancy.

   D mucoepidermoid tumours are common in elderly males and may be bilateral.

   E adenoid cystic carcinomas are aggressive tumours with a propensity for early widespread dissemination.

(Answers overleaf)

166 **A** **True**   These congenital swellings result from failed fusion of the first and second pharyngeal arches.

B **False**   The anterior border of the upper third is the classical site.

C **True**

D **True**   This is the classical site for a branchial fistula.

E **True**   The fistulous tract extends deeply between the internal and external carotid arteries and may extend to the level of the anterior pillar of the palatine tonsil. This tract requires to be completely excised to avoid recurrent problems.

167 **A** **True**   The peak incidence for benign tumours is in the sixth decade, and in the seventh decade for malignant tumours.

B **False**   Over 80% of all salivary tumours affect the parotid gland, and approximately 15% of these are malignant. Tumours of the minor salivary glands constitute 10% of all salivary tumours, 45% of which are malignant.

C **False**   It is virtually exclusive to the parotid gland and in 10% of cases is multifocal and/or bilateral. This is a benign tumour with a male preponderance and a peak incidence in the seventh decade.

D **False**   This tumour is classically slow growing with a propensity for invasion of the perineural lymphatics, causing pain and facial nerve involvement.

E **True**   In approximately 3% of cases. A much higher proportion of recurrent pleomorphic adenomas prove to be malignant (25%).

168 **A** **True**

B **False**   These tumours have pseudopodia which extend deeply into the gland, and therefore formal excision of the superficial portion of the gland is the treatment of choice.

C **False**   Mucoepidermoid tumours are the most common type of malignancy.

D **False**   This is a disease with a marked female proponderance and a peak incidence in the fifth decade. There is a spectrum of malignancy with a 5-year and 15-year survival rate of 80% and 70% respectively.

E **False**   These are slow growing but are resistant to treatment and have a high rate of recurrence.

(For more information, see ch 23 of Principles and Practice of Surgery)

169 Cervical lymphadenopathy:

    A is usually painless if due to malignancy.

    B necessitates careful examination of the oral cavity, pharynx and larynx.

    C may occur in gastric carcinoma.

    D is the commonest presentation of non-Hodgkin's lymphoma.

    E with a suppurative component is usually due to myco-bacterial infection.

170 These are well recognised complications following surgical procedures of the head and neck:

    A shoulder drop and weakness of the deltopectoral girdle after radical lymph node dissection of the neck.

    B sialorrhoea (dribble of saliva from the angle of the mouth) after submandibular gland excision.

    C gustatory sweating after superficial parotidectomy.

    D Horner's syndrome after total conservative parotidectomy.

    E exposure keratitis after parotid surgery.

(Answers overleaf)

169 A True Painful lesions generally have an inflammatory or infective aetiology.

B True A full ENT examination with indirect laryngoscopy is mandatory. It is also important to examine other areas for evidence of lymph node enlargement clinically and/or radiologically, i.e. chest X-ray, CT scan of abdomen.

C True Troissier's node in the left supraclavicular fossa. Breast, oesophagus, lung, ovary and testes are other common primary sites with a propensity for cervical dissemination.

D False This is a more common presentation of Hodgkin's lymphoma. Non-Hodgkin's lymphoma arises more commonly in the gastrointestinal tract or in other extranodal sites.

E False Although suppurative lymphadenitis in the cervical region was a common mode of presentation of gastrointestinal TB in the past, this is now more commonly the result of severe streptococcal tonsillar infection.

170 A True This is the result of sacrifice of the spinal accessory nerve, although in some cases it is possible to conserve the nerve.

B True This is the result of damage to the mandibular branch of the facial nerve, which supplies the orbicularis oris muscle. It is usually due to an inappropriately high incision within two finger-breadths of the mandibular ramus.

C True This is Frey's syndrome, which results from damage to the auriculotemporal nerve, which carries postganglionic fibres from the otic ganglion to the parotid gland as well as sensory fibres to the skin and sympathetic fibres to the sweat glands and cutaneous vessels.

D False For Horner's syndrome (miosis, ptosis, anhydrosis, enophthalmos) to occur, it is necessary to damage the cervical sympathetic chain or the stellate ganglion. This is not described in parotidectomy.

E True If the zygomatic branch of the facial nerve is damaged then the flaccid orbicularis oculi results in ectropion, and the cornea becomes damaged due to exposure. Lateral tarsorrhaphy is indicated.

(For more information, see ch 23 of Principles and Practice of Surgery)

18. Mouth, nose, throat and ear

171 Concerning oral infections and swellings:
A aphthous ulceration is due to vitamin C deficiency.
B angular cheilitis occurs in patients with vitamin deficiency (B_{12} or C) and mineral (e.g. iron) deficiency.
C inflammation of the oral mucosa (stomatitis) and gums (gingivitis) should be treated by broad-spectrum antibiotics.
D a ranula is a collection of fluid in a persistent thyroglossal duct.
E squamous papillomas on the inside of the cheek are associated with a high risk of malignant change.

172 Oral candidiasis:
A appears as a punctate yellowish rash.
B occurs most commonly underneath dentures.
C should be treated with broad-spectrum antibiotics.
D is diagnosed by taking swabs for culture.
E may be associated with oesophageal candidiasis.

173 Leukoplakia:
A refers to a 'white patch' within the mouth.
B consists of histological areas of hyperkeratosis.
C progresses to malignant change in 70% of patients.
D is associated with chronic irritation, particularly from tobacco and alcohol.
E should be treated by excision if red areas develop.

(Answers overleaf)

171 A False The aetiology of aphthous ulcers is unknown. They are common in normal individuals and are also seen in patients with Crohn's disease or ulcerative colitis.

B True Angular cheilitis (cracking at the angles of the mouth) may also be associated with dryness of the lips, cheeks and tongue.

C False Antibiotics are rarely indicated. Treatment consists of attention to oral hygiene and correction of precipitating causes such as dehydration, febrile illness and malnourishment.

D False A ranula is a retention cyst of mucus or accessory salivary glands, situated under the tongue.

E False They are common and may be multiple but they never become malignant.

172 A False The classical appearance is a whitish membrane which resembles milk curds.

B True In debilitated patients it may occur anywhere in the mouth, particularly the palate, fauces, tongue and hypopharynx.

C False It is often associated with inappropriate broad-spectrum antibiotic therapy. Treatment consists of topical nystatin lozenges or suspensions and improvement of oral hygiene and general health.

D False The diagnosis is confirmed by taking scrapings for microscopic examination.

E True Particularly in severely ill or debilitated patients and also in association with inappropriate broad-spectrum antibiotic use.

173 A True It occurs most commonly on the tongue and buccal mucosa.

B True In some areas, dysplasia may also occur.

C False This occurs in 10% of patients (particularly those with dysplasia).

D True It usually regresses with attention to oral hygiene and abstinence from tobacco and alcohol.

E True This is known as erythroplakia and is associated with a high incidence of dysplasia (70%) and malignant change.

(For more information, see ch 24 of Principles and Practice of Surgery)

174 Concerning cancer of the tongue and oral cavity:
A chronic oral sepsis is the major aetiological factor.
B it is commoner in females than in males.
C it occurs most often in patients over 70 years of age.
D it usually presents with a painful ulcer.
E it is usually unresponsive to radiotherapy.

175 Concerning infectious conditions of the oropharynx:
A acute pharyngitis is usually due to a bacterial infection.
B acute tonsillitis is caused by staphylococcal infection.
C peritonsillar abscess (quinsy) should be treated by antibiotics.
D retropharyngeal abscess usually occurs secondary to an upper respiratory infection in children and adults.
E bilateral cervical lymph node enlargement in an adolescent or young adult may be due to Epstein–Barr virus infection.

176 Concerning disorders of the hypopharynx:
A tumours in this region are usually squamous cell carcinomas.
B the first manifestation of malignant disease in this region may be cervical lymph node enlargement.
C treatment of pharyngeal tumours usually involves surgical excision and adjuvant radiotherapy.
D a pharyngeal pouch is due to mucosal herniation between the cricopharyngeus muscle and the muscle of the oesophagus.
E treatment of a pharyngeal pouch consists of excision of the pouch, repair of the deficit and division of the cricopharyngeus muscle (myotomy) below the defect.

177 The following are causes of vocal cord paralysis:
A apical lung carcinoma (Pancoast tumour) on the left side.
B surgical trauma during thyroidectomy.
C pulmonary tuberculosis.
D Guillain–Barré syndrome.
E aortic aneurysm.

(Answers overleaf)

174 A False Tobacco smoking is the major aetiological factor.
  B False It is more common in males.
  C True   It is rare before the age of 45.
  D False It is usually painless, thus patients tend to present late.
  E False For small lesions, surgery and radiotherapy are equally effective. Treatment of large lesions, with or without node involvement, usually involves surgery, with or without radiotherapy.

175 A False It is usually due to a viral infection.
  B False It is due to β-haemolytic streptococci.
  C False As with any localised collection of pus, it should be treated by incision and drainage.
  D False This is true in children — in adults it is usually secondary to tuberculosis of the spine.
  E True   Infectious mononucleosis (glandular fever).

176 A True
  B True   In particular, lesions of the pyriform fossa may become quite large before causing local symptoms and may present with cervical node enlargement. Thus, in patients with cervical node enlargement, primary pathology in the hypopharynx must always be excluded.
  C True
  D False It is due to herniation between the lower pharyngeal muscles, thyropharyngeus and cricopharyngeus (Killian's dehiscence).
  E True

177 A True   Due to involvement of the left recurrent laryngeal nerve.
  B True   Due to trauma to the recurrent laryngeal nerves.
  C True   Due to mediastinal lymphadenopathy.
  D True   Due to peripheral neuropathy affecting the vagus or recurrent laryngeal nerves.
  E True   Due to stretching of the left recurrent laryngeal nerve.

(For more information, see ch 24 of Principles and Practice of Surgery)

178 Concerning laryngeal tumours:
A the majority occur on the glottis.
B adult papillomas are usually multiple.
C the most frequent presenting symptom is hoarseness.
D laryngeal carcinoma frequently metastasises to distant sites.
E laryngeal carcinoma is invariably inoperable by the time of diagnosis.

179 Acute otitis media:
A occurs most commonly in children.
B is usually due to a viral infection.
C should be treated by analgesia and antibiotics.
D may be associated with a conductive-type hearing loss.
E in an adult, may be associated with nasopharyngeal carcinoma.

180 Sensorineural hearing loss may be due to:
A hereditary deafness.
B rubella.
C cyclosporin antibiotics.
D meningitis.
E presbycusis.

(Answers overleaf)

178 A True And can thus be detected by indirect laryngoscopy (indicated in all patients who are hoarse for more than 3 weeks).

B False They are usually single and do not recur following excision.

C True Stridor is also an important presenting symptom.

D False Distant metastases are rare but, with large tumours, cervical lymph node metastases are frequent.

E False Up to 95% of patients can be treated, many with a hope of cure. Treatment consists of radiotherapy followed by laryngectomy in patients with residual or recurrent disease.

179 A True

B False Usually due to bacterial infection (pneumococcus, streptococcus, and *H. influenzae*).

C True Occasionally, myringotomy may be indicated.

D True

E True

180 A True

B True

C False But it may occur with aminoglycoside antibiotics.

D True

E True Analogous to presbyopia, where normal hearing declines progressively after the age of 40.

(For more information, see ch 24 of Principles and Practice of Surgery)

19. Abdomen, abdominal wall and hernia

181 Ascites:

A is described as a transudate if the protein concentration is greater than 25 g/l.

B occurs as a transudate in tuberculous peritonitis.

C if blood-stained, suggests the presence of infection.

D is most commonly clear and straw-coloured.

E is commonly caused by cirrhotic portal hypertension.

182 Ascites:

A is demonstrated clinically by 'shifting dullness'.

B may be associated with umbilical herniation.

C may be treated with diuretics.

D may be treated with a peritoneovenous shunt.

E can be treated very safely by regular paracentesis.

183 Concerning lesions of the abdominal wall:

A a patent communication may be present between the ileum and the umbilicus.

B metastatic carcinoma may present in the umbilicus.

C isolated rectus sheath haematoma may occur.

D a desmoid tumour may arise in the rectus muscle.

E a urinary fistula to the umbilicus may occur.

(Answers overleaf)

181 **A False** This is an exudate; a transudate has a protein concentration of less than 25 g/l.
    B False In this case the protein concentration is very high (exudate); this also occurs with bacterial peritonitis and acute pancreatitis, i.e. in situations associated with inflammation of the peritoneum. In other situations (e.g. uncomplicated liver cirrhosis), the ascites is a transudate.
    C False This suggests the presence of malignancy — infected ascites is usually cloudy.
    D True As, for example, in liver disease.
    E True

182 **A True** This is the best physical sign — the demarcation line between flank dullness and anterior resonance shifts posteriorly as the patient moves away from the side being examined.
    B True Raised intra-abdominal pressure causes eversion and herniation at the umbilicus.
    C True For example, spironolactone, used to counteract the secondary hyperaldosteronism which occurs in cirrhotic liver disease.
    D True Used in chronic cases; examples include the Le Veen and Denver shunts which direct ascitic fluid via a one-way valve from the peritoneal cavity to the internal jugular vein.
    E False Regular paracentesis will inevitably result in secondary bacterial infection.

183 **A True** This occurs in association with a persistent vitello-intestinal duct and Meckel's diverticulum. It results in a red, discharging lesion at the umbilicus ('strawberry tumour').
    B True Secondary to intra-abdominal carcinoma, producing a firm nodule at the umbilicus ('Sister Joseph's nodule').
    C True Due to rupture of the inferior epigastric artery, usually in patients with chronic cough.
    D True From the fibrous intermuscular septae. It may be associated with intestinal polyposis in Gardner's syndrome.
    E True Due to persistence of the urachus.

(For more information, see ch 25 of Principles and Practice of Surgery)

184 Femoral hernias:
  A occur more commonly in females.
  B are the commonest type of groin hernia in females.
  C project through the femoral canal which is bordered medially by the femoral vein.
  D rarely become strangulated.
  E clinically, present as a bulge on the upper lateral aspect of the thigh.

185 Inguinal hernias:
  A if indirect, enter the deep inguinal ring medial to the inferior epigastric vessels.
  B if direct, exit the peritoneal cavity between the rectus muscle, the inguinal ligament and the inferior epigastric artery.
  C if indirect, exit the inguinal canal lateral to the pubic tubercle.
  D if direct, occur as a result of persistence of the processus vaginalis.
  E occur most commonly in males.

186 Concerning the difference between direct and indirect inguinal hernias:
  A direct are the most common type.
  B it is easy to distinguish between the two, clinically.
  C pressure over the deep inguinal ring will control an indirect hernia when the patient coughs.
  D indirect are more likely to become irreducible and undergo strangulation.
  E direct occur in infants.

187 Complications of groin hernias include:
  A irreducibility.
  B obstruction.
  C strangulation.
  D strangulation of the colon.
  E gangrene of the skin.

(Answers overleaf)

184 **A** **True**
　　B **False** Although femoral hernias are found more commonly in females than in males, the indirect inguinal hernia is still the most common groin hernia.
　　C **False** The relations of the femoral canal are: anteriorly, inguinal ligament; posteriorly, pectineal ligament; medially, lacunar ligament; laterally, femoral vein.
　　D **False** Due to the tight ligamentous ring around the neck of the sac, they frequently become strangulated.
　　E **False** On the upper medial aspect of the thigh.

185 **A** **False** Lateral to these.
　　B **True** These form Hasselbach's triangle.
　　C **False** Medial to this.
　　D **False** This is true for the indirect type; the direct type forms a diffuse bulge in the medial aspect of the inguinal canal, due to weakness of the conjoint tendon.
　　E **True** 85% in males.

186 **A** **False** Indirect (60%) vs direct (25%) of all groin hernias.
　　B **False** This is often difficult, particularly in an obese patient.
　　C **True** This is the basis of the clinical test — a direct hernia will not be controlled by this and will bulge out medial to the examining fingers placed over the deep ring.
　　D **True** Because of the narrower neck.
　　E **False** Indirect occur in infants, due to persistence of the processus vaginalis.

187 **A** **True** These three complications (**A–C**) represent the
　　B **True** pathological sequence as oedema and swelling of
　　C **True** the contents of the hernial sac occur, due to constriction by a tight neck of the sac.
　　D **True** Caecum on the right side, sigmoid colon on the left. The commonest contents of a groin hernial sac are omentum and small bowel, but colon, appendix, broad ligament, ovary, bladder or Meckel's diverticulum may also be found.
　　E **True** This is rare but may occur with strangulation, bowel perforation and secondary sepsis.

(For more information, see ch 25 of Principles and Practice of Surgery)

188   Rare types of hernia include:

A a sliding hernia, in which a partly peritonealised organ such as the caecum or bladder prolapses into the hernia and forms part of the sac wall.

B a Richter's hernia, in which only part of the circumference of the bowel herniates through the neck of the sac.

C a Littre's hernia, in which a Meckel's diverticulum enters the hernial sac.

D a Madyl's hernia, in which two or more loops of bowel enter the hernial sac.

E a Spigelian hernia, which occurs at the medial border of the rectus muscle.

189   Concerning abdominal wall hernias:

A a para-umbilical hernia occurs most commonly in children.

B an umbilical hernia does not usually require surgical treatment.

C incisional hernias most commonly involve transverse wounds.

D herniation does not occur through the posterior abdominal wall.

E incisional hernias often become strangulated.

190   Concerning repair of a groin hernia:

A it may be performed laparoscopically.

B a technique in which nonabsorbable mesh is placed anteriorly over the hernial defect may be used.

C recurrence will not occur if a meticulous surgical technique is used.

D in children, repair of the posterior wall of the inguinal canal is necessary.

E it may be performed as a day case.

(Answers overleaf)

188 **A** **True**
    B **True**   This is the definition of a Richter's hernia, hence it can become strangulated but not necessarily obstructed as the lumen may not be completely occluded.
    C **True**
    D **True**
    E **False**   A Spigelian hernia is a rare form of interparietal hernia which occurs at the lateral border of the rectus muscle, at the arcuate line.

189 **A** **False**   It occurs most commonly in adults and represents a hernia through the linea alba, adjacent to the umbilicus.
    B **True**   This occurs in infants, due to failure of closure of the umbilicus. The vast majority close spontaneously but if this does not occur by the age of 2, surgical closure is indicated.
    C **False**   They most commonly involve midline, vertical wounds.
    D **False**   An example of a posterior hernia is the lumbar hernia through the triangle of Petit, bounded by the spine, the posterior iliac crest and the latissimus dorsi muscle.
    E **False**   They usually have a wide neck and strangulation is not common.

190 **A** **True**   A sheet of mesh is placed over the abdominal wall defect and covered by peritoneum.
    B **True**   This is the Lichtenstein tension-free mesh repair.
    C **False**   All repair techniques have an associated recurrence rate, though this is generally very low if a meticulous surgical technique is used.
    D **False**   Treatment in children involves simple ligation of the hernial sac (herniotomy). Herniotomy plus repair of the posterior wall (herniorraphy) is performed in adults.
    E **True**   Virtually all herniotomies in children, and an increasing number of hernia repairs in adults, are performed as day cases.

(For more information, see ch 25 of Principles and Practice of Surgery)

20. The acute abdomen

191 Concerning abdominal pain:

A pain due to disease in the stomach is experienced initially in the periumbilical area.

B pain due to obstruction of the ileum is experienced initially in the periumbilical area.

C pain due to biliary colic is usually experienced in the right upper quadrant.

D pain due to cholecystitis may be experienced in the right shoulder.

E pain of renal origin does not usually 'cross' the midline.

192 Concerning abdominal pain:

A in the vast majority (>85%) of acute surgical admissions for abdominal pain, a specific cause is found.

B pain due to a vascular catastrophe (e.g. aortic aneurysm rupture) usually commences gradually and worsens progressively.

C resolution of pain usually suggests that the causative condition has resolved.

D the causative pathology may not be within the abdomen.

E pain due to peritonitis typically commences gradually and worsens progressively.

193 Concerning examination of the acute abdomen:

A Murphy's sign is a reliable sign of acute appendicitis.

B Rovsing's sign is a reliable sign of acute appendicitis.

C rebound tenderness indicates the presence of visceral peritonitis.

D cutaneous hyperaesthesia may occur over an area of inflamed parietal peritoneum.

E rectal examination should always be performed.

(Answers overleaf)

191 **A** **False** It is experienced initially in the epigastric area.
     B **True**
     C **False** The key to understanding this concept is that pain from disease of a visceral organ (visceral pain) is relatively nonspecific but is experienced in the representative area for that part of the alimentary tract — i.e. foregut pain, epigastrium; midgut pain, periumbilical area; hindgut pain, suprapubic area. When the pathological process extends to involve the parietal peritoneum, the pain (somatic pain) becomes more localised. Biliary colic is caused by contraction of the biliary system around a stone and is therefore visceral pain, hence is experienced in the foregut area — the epigastrium.
     D **True** Classical referred pain.
     E **True**

192 **A** **False** In 40–50% of cases, no specific cause is found, the final coded diagnosis being 'nonspecific abdominal pain'.
     B **False** A vascular catastrophe or perforation of a hollow viscus usually presents suddenly with excruciating pain.
     C **False** For example, the pain of mesenteric vascular occlusion may decrease as the bowel becomes gangrenous.
     D **True** For example, pain due to torsion of the testicle may initially be experienced in the abdomen due to the shared nerve supply (T10).
     E **True**

193 **A** **False** Acute cholecystitis.
     B **False** In acute appendicitis, deep palpation in the left iliac fossa is said to cause pain in the right iliac fossa — Rovsing's sign. However, it is a very variable and unreliable sign.
     C **False** It indicates parietal peritonitis. In this sign, pain increases sharply as the examining hand is removed quickly after deep palpation.
     D **True** However, this test is rarely useful.
     E **True** Because pelvic peritonitis may produce little abdominal tenderness, but marked tenderness on rectal examination.

(For more information, see ch 26 of Principles and Practice of Surgery)

194 Investigations in a patient presenting with an acute abdomen which are likely to be useful in the early assessment include:
A a full blood count.
B urea and electrolyte estimation.
C liver function tests.
D urinalysis.
E serum amylase.

195 Concerning investigation of the acute abdomen:
A an abdominal X-ray yields useful information in the majority of patients.
B peritoneal lavage is a useful investigation in patients with suspected peritonitis.
C laparoscopy is a useful diagnostic technique.
D ultrasonography is frequently useful.
E an abdominal X-ray will detect gallstones in the majority of patients in whom these are present.

196 Common causes of an acute abdomen include:
A appendicitis.
B ruptured Graafian follicle.
C Meckel's diverticulum.
D cholecystitis.
E acute pancreatitis.

197 In a typical case of acute generalised peritonitis:
A there is abdominal tenderness and guarding.
B there is tenderness on rectal examination.
C there is likely to be a normal extracellular fluid volume.
D a bradycardia is present.
E bowel sounds are absent.

(Answers overleaf)

194 A True   Leucocytosis is usually present in cases of acute
                     peritonitis but the white cell count is often normal
                     in the early stages.
    B True   These are essential to assess fluid and electrolyte
                     balance and requirements.
    C False   These rarely influence the emergency assessment
                     and management.
    D True   This may reveal sugar and ketones in undiagnosed
                     diabetes or diabetic ketoacidosis (which may be
                     associated with abdominal pain). It may also reveal
                     pus cells and bacteria in a urinary tract infection
                     and haematuria in patients with renal colic.
    E True   This may diagnose acute pancreatitis.

195 A False   It is useful when intestinal obstruction or
                     perforation of a viscus is suspected, but in the
                     majority of cases of acute abdomen (e.g.
                     appendicitis or cholecystitis), it is not indicated.
    B False   It is useful to assess the need for surgery in blunt
                     abdominal trauma but is rarely used to evaluate the
                     acute abdomen.
    C True   It is used increasingly to diagnose, and treat, acute
                     conditions such as appendicitis, salpingitis and
                     perforated peptic ulcer.
    D True   For example, when biliary tract disease, aortic
                     aneurysm or ovarian pathology is suspected.
    E False   Only 10% of gallstones are radio-opaque, as
                     opposed to 90% of renal stones.

196 A True   Approximately 20–25% of cases.
    B True   This produces mid-cycle pain. Pain in the later
                     stages of the menstrual cycle may be due to
                     bleeding from the corpus luteum.
    C False   This is rare.
    D True
    E False   This is certainly a cause of an acute abdomen but it
                     is relatively rare (2–3% of all admissions for acute
                     abdomen).

197 A True   Very rarely; for example, in a patient on steroids,
                     tenderness and guarding may be absent.
    B True   Especially at the anterior aspect.
    C False   There is usually a depletion of extracellular fluid
                     because of vomiting and because the normal oral
                     intake of fluid has stopped.
    D False   The pulse is usually rapid and thready, due to
                     septicaemia and dehydration.
    E True   This is usually the case, due to intestinal ileus.
                     Occasionally, bowel sounds may be heard due to
                     fluid trickling from one distended loop to another.

(For more information, see ch 26 of Principles and Practice of Surgery)

198   Treatment of acute generalised peritonitis involves:

A   intravenous fluids.
B   central vein cannulation.
C   intravenous antibiotics.
D   urinary catheterisation.
E   prompt laparotomy.

199   Concerning the acute abdomen in infants and young children:

A   intussusception is a more frequent cause than in adults.
B   'medical' causes are less frequent than in adults.
C   appendicitis is unusual under the age of 2 years.
D   perforated appendicitis is more frequent in children than in adults.
E   primary peritonitis occurs more frequently in adults than in children.

200   Concerning the acute abdomen in pregnancy:

A   ectopic pregnancy usually presents with vague lower abdominal/pelvic pain and a palpable mass.
B   ectopic pregnancy should be treated urgently by salpingectomy.
C   abortion is a frequent cause of a patient presenting with an acute abdomen.
D   a slight leucocytosis is a good indicator of the presence of sepsis.
E   abdominal pain is frequently due to urinary infection.

(Answers overleaf)

198 A True   To correct the fluid deficit.
    B True   CVP monitoring facilitates fluid resuscitation and helps prevent excess administration with overload, which can occur, particularly in elderly patients.
    C True   Metronidazole (against anaerobes) and a second or third generation cephalosporin (against aerobes) are generally used.
    D True   Measurement of hourly urine volume is a valuable guide to the adequacy of resuscitation.
    E True   This is a surgical emergency. There is no place for conservative management. In some centres, laparoscopy is performed initially.

199 A True   60% of cases occur between 4 and 12 months of age.
    B False   Several medical conditions, including diabetes, acute glomerulonephritis, hepatitis and meningitis present with abdominal pain more frequently in children than in adults.
    C True
    D True   Examination and assessment of a child are more difficult, resulting in delayed diagnosis.
    E False   Primary peritonitis is an unusual condition, usually confined to girls below the age of 8. It is thought to be due to retrograde infection via the genital tract. It is usually diagnosed at appendicectomy when a green or yellow sticky pus is found in the pelvis. Culture often yields *Strep. pneumoniae*. Treatment is with penicillin.

200 A False   It typically presents 7–8 weeks after the last normal period with sudden, severe abdominal pain.
    B True
    C False   It is rare for abortion to present like this. However, a septic abortion may be associated with severe lower abdominal peritonitis.
    D False   In pregnancy there is a normal physiological leucocytosis.
    E True

(For more information, see ch 26 of Principles and Practice of Surgery)

21. The oesophagus

201 The oesophagus:
   A has a definite anatomical upper sphincter.
   B has a definite anatomical lower sphincter.
   C represents a site of portal–systemic anastomosis.
   D has no sensory nerve supply to the mucosa.
   E is lined predominantly by columnar epithelium.

202 Appropriate investigations in oesophageal disease include:
   A chest X-ray.
   B barium swallow.
   C endoscopy.
   D manometry.
   E pH measurement.

203 Achalasia:
   A is due to loss of muscle tone in the lower oesophageal sphincter.
   B presents principally with gastro-oesophageal reflux and heartburn.
   C may result in aspiration pneumonitis.
   D may be treated by hydrostatic balloon dilatation.
   E is associated with an increased risk of development of oesophageal carcinoma.

204 Gastro-oesophageal reflux:
   A occurs only when a hiatus hernia is present.
   B may predispose to stricture development.
   C may predispose to development of Barrett's oesophagus.
   D usually requires surgical treatment.
   E may be treated surgically by gastropexy.

(Answers overleaf)

201 **A** **True** Formed by the cricopharyngeus muscle.

B **False** This cannot be defined anatomically but consists of a 3–5 cm long high pressure area which is tonically 'closed' at rest and prevents gastro-oesophageal reflux.

C **True** Between the left gastric veins and the azygous venous system at the lower end — the site where oesophageal varices may develop.

D **False** Various symptoms, including heartburn, are mediated via sensory nerve endings in the mucosa.

E **False** It is lined predominantly by squamous epithelium, apart from the distal 1–2 cm where the epithelium is columnar.

202 **A** **True** Swallowed foreign bodies or a large intrathoracic hiatus hernia may be seen (a hiatus hernia may contain air/fluid level).

B **True** This may demonstrate structural abnormalities such as tumours, strictures or diverticulae, and functional disorders such as achalasia.

C **True** This may be performed by flexible or rigid methods.

D **True** Used to assess motility disorders such as achalasia.

E **True** Usually monitored over a 24-hour period, to detect gastro-oesophageal reflux.

203 **A** **False** There is spasm of this sphincter, producing a functional obstruction.

B **False** The cardinal symptom is dysphagia.

C **True** Food regurgitation and aspiration may occur, for example, when the patient is asleep.

D **True** If this fails, a cardiomyotomy (Heller's procedure) may be necessary.

E **True**

204 **A** **False** It may occur in the absence of a hiatus hernia.

B **True** Particularly when there is marked oesophagitis and ulceration.

C **True** In this condition, persistent reflux and oesophagitis lead to metaplasia of the squamous epithelium, in which there is an increased incidence of carcinoma developing.

D **False** In the majority of patients symptoms can be controlled by medical therapy (e.g. H_2 receptor antagonists or proton pump inhibitors).

E **False** Surgical treatment involves a fundoplication. For example, Nissen fundoplication, in which the fundus of the stomach is wrapped around the lower oesophagus so that when an increase in intragastric pressure occurs it compresses and occludes the enclosed oesophagus.

(For more information, see ch 27 of Principles and Practice of Surgery)

205 Concerning hiatus hernia:
  A the rolling type is the most common.
  B the rolling type usually presents with gastro-oesophageal reflux.
  C the sliding type is usually associated with gastro-oesophageal reflux and heartburn.
  D the rolling type requires surgical treatment.
  E the sliding type may be diagnosed on chest X-ray.

206 Premalignant conditions of the oesophagus include:
  A achalasia.
  B candida infection.
  C Plummer–Vinson syndrome.
  D Barrett's oesophagus.
  E corrosive stricture.

207 The following are recognised conditions of the oesophagus:
  A Boerhaave's syndrome.
  B familial oesophageal cancer in association with hyperkeratosis of the palms and soles.
  C Crohn's disease.
  D Mallory–Weiss syndrome.
  E Zenker's diverticulum.

208 Aetiological factors in carcinoma of the oesophagus include:
  A smoking.
  B alcohol.
  C lower socio-economic groups.
  D female sex.
  E pharyngeal pouch (Zenker's diverticulum).

(Answers overleaf)

205 **A** **False** Sliding hiatus hernia is much more common (95% of cases).
  B **False** It usually presents with chest pain and dysphagia due to distension of the intrathoracic stomach and compression of the oesophagus.
  C **False** The majority of patients with a sliding hiatus hernia have no symptoms.
  D **True** Surgery is always indicated because of the risk of strangulation of the intrathoracic stomach.
  E **False** The rolling type may be demonstrated by visualisation of a shadow, with or without a fluid level, in the posterior mediastinum.

206 **A** **True**
  B **False**
  C **True** Associated with a post-cricoid web.
  D **True**
  E **True**

207 **A** **True** Describes spontaneous rupture of the lower oesophagus following forcible vomiting and retching.
  B **True** Hyperkeratosis of the palms and soles is known as tylosis.
  C **True** Although it is extremely rare in this site.
  D **True** Describes a linear mucosal tear in the lower oesophagus, associated with vomiting. It presents with haematemesis and later melaena.
  E **True** This is a pharyngeal pouch which presents between the cricopharyngeus and thyropharyngeus muscles (Killian's dehiscence).

208 **A** **True** Most patients in the Western world developing oesophageal cancer are heavy smokers.
  B **True**
  C **True** This may reflect increased cigarette smoking or dietary deficiencies.
  D **False** In the UK, the male-to-female ratio is 1.5:1.
  E **True**

(For more information, see ch 27 of Principles and Practice of Surgery)

209   Carcinoma of the oesophagus:

   A is usually an adenocarcinoma.
   B often presents with bleeding.
   C typically presents with progressive dysphagia and weight loss.
   D frequently invades adjacent structures.
   E is associated with a prognosis similar to colorectal carcinoma.

210   Concerning treatment of oesophageal carcinoma:

   A adenocarcinomas are usually sensitive to radiotherapy.
   B carcinoma of the upper third is generally treated by radiotherapy.
   C CT scanning of the chest and abdomen should be performed.
   D palliative relief of dysphagia may be achieved by dilatation and insertion of a rigid tube.
   E the presence of hoarseness is a sign of unresectable disease.

(Answers overleaf)

209 **A False**   More than 90% are squamous carcinomas.
Adenocarcinomas can arise from the columnar
epithelium in the lower third of the oesophagus.

    B False   This is a surprisingly uncommon initial mode of
presentation.

    C True

    D True   Erosion into the bronchus may produce a
broncho-oesophageal fistula, and erosion of the
recurrent laryngeal nerve may produce hoarseness.

    E False   The prognosis is much worse for oesophageal
carcinoma, the overall 5-year survival rate being
5–10%.

210 **A False**   Squamous carcinomas may be radiosensitive but
adenocarcinomas are not.

    B True

    C True   To detect mediastinal or hepatic involvement.

    D True   Examples include the Celestin and Nottingham
tubes. Alternatively, repeated laser photo-
coagulation may be used to maintain the lumen.

    E True   This indicates mediastinal invasion.

(For more information, see ch 27 of Principles and Practice of Surgery)

22. Gastroduodenal disorders

211 Aetiological factors in peptic ulceration include:
- **A** *Helicobacter pylori* infection.
- **B** high intragastric pH.
- **C** burn injury.
- **D** Zollinger–Ellison syndrome.
- **E** bile reflux.

212 Current medical therapy for peptic ulceration includes:
- **A** H_2-receptor antagonists.
- **B** antibiotics.
- **C** H^+K^+ ATPase inhibition.
- **D** prostaglandin antagonists.
- **E** anticholinergic drugs to block gastric acid secretion.

213 Complications of duodenal ulcer include:
- **A** bleeding.
- **B** perforation.
- **C** malignant change.
- **D** dumping.
- **E** stricture formation

214 Surgical procedures currently used for duodenal ulcer include:
- **A** highly selective vagotomy.
- **B** selective vagotomy.
- **C** truncal vagotomy and antrectomy.
- **D** laparoscopic vagotomy.
- **E** vagotomy plus gastroenterostomy.

(Answers overleaf)

211 A True   Although the mechanism is uncertain.
   B False   Peptic ulceration is associated with high intragastric acidity and low pH.
   C True   This may result in duodenal stress ulceration or erosions known as Curling's ulcers.
   D True   Excess acidity occurs in association with hypergastrinaemia due to G-cell hyperplasia of the antrum or a gastrin-producing tumour of the pancreas or duodenum.
   E True   This may damage the gastric mucosa.

212 A True
   B True   For eradication of *Helicobacter pylori*.
   C True   Otherwise known as proton pump inhibition.
   D False   These are associated with peptic ulceration. Prostaglandin analogues such as misoprostil may be used.
   E False   The side effects associated with these are significant and they are no longer used.

213 A True   Usually due to erosion of the gastroduodenal artery by a posterior ulcer. This may be treated by endoscopic adrenaline or sclerosant injection but may require surgical suture-ligation and vagotomy.
   B True   Usually of an anterior ulcer. This may be treated by open or laparoscopic closure of the perforation.
   C False   This may occur with gastric ulcers. Hence the follow-up of patients with duodenal ulcer is 'symptomatic' but that of gastric ulcer must include check endoscopy to exclude malignancy.
   D False   But this may be a complication of some forms of surgical treatment.
   E True   Usually associated with chronic ulceration, leading to pyloric stenosis.

214 A True   This has the advantage of denervating the acid-producing area but not the pylorus. Therefore, a drainage operation such as pyloroplasty or gastroenterostomy is not necessary.
   B False   No longer widely used.
   C True   This represents the maximal way to decrease gastric acidity — by denervating the stomach and removing the acid-producing area. It was used principally for treatment of recurrent, intractable ulceration but, with modern medical therapy, is now rarely required.
   D True
   E True   Used principally for treatment of pyloric stenosis.

(For more information, see ch 28 of Principles and Practice of Surgery)

215 Concerning complications of surgery for peptic ulceration:

A bile vomiting may occur.
B diarrhoea may occur.
C dumping may occur.
D dumping, diarrhoea and bile vomiting often occur following highly selective vagotomy.
E reactive hypoglycaemia may occur.

216 The following statements are true:

A the risk of recurrent bleeding following surgery for a bleeding peptic ulcer may be reduced by using intravenous H_2-receptor antagonists.
B the risk of recurrent bleeding following surgery for a bleeding peptic ulcer may be reduced by addition of a vagotomy at the time of surgery.
C the incidence of duodenal ulceration in the UK is decreasing.
D peptic ulceration may occur in the oesophagus.
E a barium meal is the most accurate diagnostic test for gastric or duodenal ulceration.

217 Zollinger–Ellison syndrome:

A is associated with hypogastrinaemia.
B may be due to a gastrinoma, the majority of which are benign.
C is characterised by ulceration which classically involves one site.
D is often associated with diarrhoea.
E may be associated with other endocrine abnormalities.

(Answers overleaf)

215 A True   **A, B** and **C** may occur if the normal pyloric control
B True   of gastric emptying is destroyed and the gastric
C True   outlet sphincter is rendered 'incontinent'.
D False   In this operation the pyloric mechanism is left
        intact. The complications may occur following
        pyloroplasty, gastroenterostomy or gastric
        resection.
E True   This was once known as 'late' dumping. Symptoms
        are due to rapid absorption of glucose from the
        upper small bowel and reactive excessive insulin
        secretion, with resultant hypoglycaemia.

216 A False Although they are widely used in this situation,
        clinical trials have shown that H_2-receptor
        antagonists do not prevent recurrent bleeding.
B True
C True   The decrease in incidence of this disease predated
        the introduction of H_2-receptor antagonists or other
        medical therapies.
D True   The duodenum and stomach are the common sites
        but it may also occur in the oesophagus, jejunum
        (in the Zollinger–Ellison syndrome) and terminal
        ileum (in a Meckel's diverticulum).
E False   Barium meal has been replaced by endoscopy
        which is more accurate, particularly for superficial
        erosions, and also allows biopsy of gastric ulcers
        to exclude malignancy and to test for *Helicobacter
        pylori*.

217 A False Hypergastrinaemia and associated fulminant peptic
        ulceration.
B False   Two-thirds of gastrinomas are malignant and more
        than three-quarters of patients have multiple
        tumours.
C False   Ulceration often occurs at multiple sites in the
        stomach, duodenum or jejunum.
D True   Due to a combination of jejunitis and steatorrhoea
        caused by destruction of lipase by acid.
E True   As part of a multiple endocrine neoplasia (MENI)
        syndrome.

(For more information, see ch 28 of Principles and Practice of Surgery)

218 The following statements are true:
 A Ménétriers's disease is characterised by atrophy of the gastric mucosa.
 B most swallowed foreign bodies fail to pass beyond the pylorus.
 C stress ulceration associated with burns, severe trauma or multiple organ failure characteristically involves the duodenum.
 D a Billroth I gastrectomy involves anastomosis of the proximal gastric remnant to the proximal jejunum.
 E hypertrophic pyloric stenosis classically occurs in children aged 1–2 years.

219 Aetiological factors in gastric adenocarcinoma include:
 A blood group O.
 B previous gastric resection.
 C chronic gastritis.
 D higher socio-economic groups.
 E gastric polyps.

220 Gastric cancer:
 A is always an adenocarcinoma.
 B may spread diffusely along the stomach wall.
 C may metastasise to the ovaries.
 D usually presents at a late stage in the disease.
 E can usually be treated by a potentially curative resection.

(Answers overleaf)

218 A False This disease, of unknown origin, is characterised by giant hypertrophy of the mucosal rugal folds. Protein loss from this may result in a low plasma albumin and peripheral oedema.

B False Most pass through the gastrointestinal tract and surgery is usually not necessary.

C False It involves the proximal stomach — the area lined by acid secreting mucosa. Stress ulceration associated with closed head injury characteristically involves the duodenum.

D False This describes the Billroth II or Polya gastrectomy. In the Billroth I gastrectomy, the proximal gastric remnant is anastomosed to the duodenum.

E False It classically occurs in infants and presents with vomiting and a palpable abdominal mass when the infant is feeding. It is treated by longitudinal division of the hypertrophed pyloric muscle (Ramstedt's operation).

219 A False Blood group A.

B True Particularly surgery performed for gastric ulcer; the risk increases with decreasing age at the time of operation. Nowadays, however, gastric resection for treatment of peptic ulcer is becoming less frequent.

C True This is commonly found in association with atrophy of the mucosa, achlorhydria, pernicious anaemia and intestinal metaplasia.

D False Gastric carcinoma occurs more frequently in lower socio-economic groups, although this may reflect a higher incidence of cigarette smoking.

E True Adenomatous gastric polyps may occur (although much less frequently than colonic polyps) and, particularly if greater than 2 cm in diameter, are associated with a high incidence of malignant change.

220 A False It is almost always an adenocarcinoma, but lymphoma and leiomyosarcoma also occur.

B True Producing the so-called 'leather bottle stomach' (linitis plastica).

C True By transcoelomic spread — Krükenberg tumour. Spread via this route may also result in metastases in the peritoneum, omentum and rectovesical pouch.

D True Although in some countries (e.g. Japan) it is detected at an early stage by aggressive screening (early gastric cancer) and treatment is associated with a much better prognosis.

E False In many cases the disease is advanced at the time of presentation and only a palliative bypass (e.g. gastroenterostomy) is appropriate.

(For more information, see ch 28 of Principles and Practice of Surgery)

23. The appendix

Intestinal obstruction

221 The vermiform appendix:
  A develops as a conical diverticulum from the dependent pole of the caecum.
  B is the embryological remnant of the vitello-intestinal duct.
  C marks the exact midpoint of the gastrointestinal tract.
  D receives a tenuous blood supply from the right colic artery.
  E is located at laparotomy by following the taeniae coli which converge on its base.

222 Acute appendicitis:
  A is the most common acute general surgical emergency.
  B is declining in incidence.
  C is uncommon in developing countries.
  D has a peak incidence in the second decade of life.
  E may occur secondary to a caecal carcinoma.

(Answers overleaf)

221 A True   The appendix initially develops from the lower pole of the caecum however with differential growth, it eventually projects from the posteromedial wall some 2 cm inferior to the ileocaecal valve.

B False   Meckel's diverticulum, which occurs 60 cm proximal to the ileocaecal valve on the antimesenteric border of the ileum, is present in 2% of the population and itself can become obstructed and mimic appendicitis. It marks the mid-point of the intestinal tract about which the anti-clockwise 270° rotation takes place in intrauterine life.

C False
D False   It receives a profuse blood supply from the ileocolic artery in the shape of one or two appendicular arteries.

E True   The appendix base is located at the confluence of the taeniae coli, which represent condensations of the longitudinal smooth muscle.

222 A True
B True   The incidence of acute appendicitis, which is influenced by dietary and genetic factors, has fallen substantially over the last 30 years. In western countries, 16% of the population undergoes appendicectomy.

C True   The incidence of appendicitis in the developing countries is increasing as these countries adopt a more refined western style diet.

D True   Although the incidence is extremely low in the extremes of life it is generally this patient groups that account for the morbidity and mortality associated with this condition.

E True   Secondary appendicitis accounts for a small proportion of cases. Primary tumours of the appendix and caecum, infantile ileocolic intussusception and parasitic infestation may cause obstruction of the lumen and consequently appendicitis.

(For more information, see chs 30 and 31 of Principles and Practice of Surgery)

223 In acute appendicitis:
- **A** obstruction of the lumen is the initiating event.
- **B** the indigenous bacterial flora are typical of the large bowel.
- **C** a faecalith is present is <10% of cases.
- **D** if untreated will invariably progress to necrosis and perforation.
- **E** prophylactic antibiotics should be administered to reduce the risk postoperative wound infection.

224 In acute appendicitis:
- **A** paraumbilical colic is usually the earliest symptom.
- **B** errors in diagnosis are most common in young women.
- **C** anorexia is almost always present.
- **D** abdominal examination remains the cornerstone of diagnosis.
- **E** investigations are of limited value and may be unnecessary.

(Answers overleaf)

223 A True   Inflammation is initiated by obstruction of the
lumen either as a result of lymphoid hyperplasia
secondary to viral infection or due to a faecolith in
the lumen. Once obstructed, the appendix distends
with secretions, resulting in mucosal necrosis and
invasion of the appendicular wall with bacteria.

B True   The appendix contains aerobic and anaerobic
bacteria typical of the indiginous colonic flora.

C False   A faecalith is present in 30–40% of resected
appendices, and gangrene is twice as common
(75–80%) in these appendices compared to those
containing no faecalith.

D False   Inflammation follows a variable pattern which may
be aborted or delayed by host defences at any time.
The perforation rate is 25% in patients with pain for
<24 hours but the rate only increases by 10% in
patients with a history for >48 hours.

E True   Three perioperative doses of 1g of metronidazole
administered rectally which is effective against
bacteroides spp. will considerably reduce the
incidence of wound infection.

224 A True   Obstruction of the appendix is the initiating event
in acute appendicitis and as the appendix is a
midgut organ, and when obstructed, it will result in
paraumbilical colic.

B True   In young women various gynaecological conditions (Mittelschmerz from rupture of the Graafian
follicle at ovulation, cyst rupture or torsion, ectopic
pregnancy and infective conditions of the adnexae)
present with lower abdominal pain and urinary
tract infections and non-specific abdominal pain
are more common in this patient population.

C True   Anorexia is one of the more consistent features of
appendicitis. Unfortunately only 50% of patients
with acute appendicitis present with classical
symptoms.

D True   The following should be sought: (1) point of
maximal tenderness over McBurney's point;
(2) muscular guarding and/or rebound tenderness;
(3) presence of a mass — this may suggest the
presence of an inflammatory mass.

E True   Economy of investigations is worthwhile, and the
diagnosis and management of the patient with
acute apendicitis can be accomplished without any
tests.

(For more information, see chs 30 and 31 of Principles and Practice of Surgery)

225   Concerning tumours of the appendix:
   A   adenocarcinomas constitute the majority of tumours.
   B   carcinoid tumours are an incidental finding in 0.5% of all
           removed appendices.
   C   carcinoid tumours should be treated by right
           hemicolectomy.
   D   may result in pseudomyxoma peritonei.
   E   may present with flushing, bronchospasm and diarrhoea.

226   Concerning intestinal obstruction:
   A   it has an associated mortality of >25%.
   B   history and examination will usually identify the site of the
           obstruction.
   C   colicky abdominal pain is characterisitic of functional
           intestinal obstruction.
   D   the presence of localised abdominal pain suggests the onset
           of strangulation.
   E   plain radiological examination will usually denote the cause
           of the obstruction.

(Answers overleaf)

225 A False Carcinoid tumors constitute approximately 85%, adenocarcinomas 14% and a small proportion are mucinous neoplasms and lymphosarcomas.

B True

C False Carcinoid tumours of the appendix are usually benign and appendicectomy is usually curative.

D True Mucocoele of the appendix may have a benign or malignant aetiology. If it occurs as the result of the rare cystadenocarcinoma, rupture of the appendix will seed the peritoneal cavity with malignant mucus secreting cells producing this debilitating condition.

E True This is the carcinoid syndrome and although extremely rare it may occur if a primary intestinal carcinoid tumour metastasises to the liver secreting 5-Hydroxytryptamine, 5-Hydroxytryptophan, kallikrein, histamine, prostaglandins or ACTH.

226 A False Intestinal obstruction accounts for approximately 3% of all emergency surgical admissions. The mortality rate in the late nineteenth century was reported as >45%, however this figure has fallen to <10% today.

B True The classical features of intestinal obstruction are: (1) crampy abdominal pain; (2) abdominal distension; (3) vomiting and (4) absolute constipation. Depending on the sequential development or predominance of one or other of these clinical features permits accurate determination of the site of the obstruction.

C False This is a feature of mechanical obstruction.The absence of pain is frequently a characteristic of a functional obstruction, i.e. ileus or pseudoobstruction.

D True Strangulation infers vascular compromise of the intestine and is usually a late manifestation of untreated intestinal obstruction. The peritoneal somatic surface becomes involved in the inflammatory process and consequently pain becomes localised.

E False The site of the obstruction can usually be confidently determined; however, the underlying diagnosis is only rarely apparent.

(For more information, see chs 30 and 31 of Principles and Practice of Surgery)

227 Pyloric outlet obstruction:
  A results in early profuse bile stained vomiting.
  B of infancy is a radiological diagnosis.
  C in adulthood is due exclusively to longstanding duodenal ulceration.
  D produces a metabolic acidosis.
  E results in an increased renal excretion of hydrogen ions.

228 Acute mechanical large bowel obstruction:
  A is more common on the left side of the colon.
  B is readily diagnosed on plain abdominal radiography.
  C due to sigmoid volvulus usually requires surgical intervention.
  D due to a carcinoma of the sigmoid colon should be treated primarily by a defunctioning loop colostomy.
  E is more hazardous in the presence of a competent ileocaecal valve.

(Answers overleaf)

227 A False A characteristic feature of pyloric outlet obstruction is the absence of bile in the vomitus. The most definitive physical finding is the presence of a succussion splash on abdominal examination.

B False This is classically diagnosed clinically by way of a test meal, although ultrasonography is being used to confirm the diagnosis. A test is positive if visible gastric peristalsis is evident, a tumour is felt in the right upper quadrant and the infant experiences projectile vomiting.

C False This is one common cause; however, it is important to exclude a primary gastric malignancy by way of endoscopic assessment and biopsy.

D False The characteristic electrolyte and acid base disturbance is a hypokalaemic, hypochloraemic metabolic alkalosis.

E True Despite the resultant alkalosis, the body's natural homeostatic principle is to conserve potassium ions at the expense of hydrogen ions, which results in an increased secretion of hydrogen ions from the renal tubules and consequently paradoxical aciduria.

228 A True Compared with the descending and sigmoid colon which have a much narrower lumen. Faeces in the descending colon is solid whilst in the right colon the faeces are fluid in consistency. Neoplasms affecting the right colon are usually polypoid, whereas those occurring on the left side are annular-constricting in nature.

B False It is impossible on plain radiography to differentiate between a functional or mechanical large bowel obstruction without the use of a contrast enema.

C False The condition has a classical radiological appearance and can be managed successfully conservatively by sigmoidoscopic decompression. Best results are obtained with the patient prone with full flexion of the hips and knees.

D False In a Hartmann's procedure colonic resection is performed the rectal stump oversewn and a temporary end colostomy fashioned in the left iliac fossa. Another option is to perform on-table colonic lavage and perform a primary anastomosis.

E True This produces an obstructed closed loop with potential caecal distension and perforation.

(For more information, see chs 30 and 31 of Principles and Practice of Surgery)

229 In intestinal obstruction:

   A dilatation is mainly the result of a failure to move the
      ingested material.
   B systemic effects are a late feature.
   C electrolyte disturbances may potentiate the obstruction.
   D the most important primary task is to remove the cause of
      the obstruction.
   E due to adhesions, the majority of the adhesions are
      congenital in origin.

230 Intestinal volvulus:

   A can affect the stomach.
   B can affect the caecum.
   C occurs most commonly in the descending colon.
   D is exclusively a disease of adulthood.
   E may have a dietary aetiology.

(Answers overleaf)

229 A False This is due to not simply the result of a failure to move the ingested material but more to swallowed air and fluid secreted into the lumen from the gastrointestinal tact. This stagnant fluid is rapidly colonised by bacteria which generate about one third of the gas in the obstructed intestine.

B False By the time of diagnosis the systemic effects are well established.

C True Although the tendancy is to preserve sodium ions, potassium losses may be extreme. Hypokalaemia will aggravate the ileus.

D False Management aims are: (1) to provide adequate resuscitation; (2) to establish whether the obstruction is functional or mechanical, identify a site and the most likely cause; (3) to arrest and reverse the associated fluid and electrolyte abnormality; (4) prevent peritoneal contamination by gastrointestinal content; (5) to remove the cause of the obstruction. (definitive surgery)

E False Approximately 90% are iatrogenic, i.e. post surgery, radiation, drugs. 10% are related to inflammatory conditions (appendicitis, diverticulitis, cholecystitis, salpingitis). Ladd's bands are congenital adhesions which are rare.

230 A True The stomach is normally well anchored, however if the points of tethering especially at the hiatus and pylorus are weakened then twisting can occur in either an organo-axial or mesenterico-axial plane. This is seen in patients with connective tissue disorders e.g. Ehlers-Danlos syndrome, or may occur secondarily to diaphragmatic herniae.

B True The caecum may be very mobile, especially in congenital 'failed caecal descent' and can twist producing intestinal obstruction. It is encountered in adult life and has the characteristic 'bird's beak' deformity on barium enema.

C False This is a retroperitoneal structure —The most common site is the sigmoid colon.

D False The process of rotation of the midgut in intrauterine life may be arrested at any stage reslting in various anomalies. The most serious occurs when the intestine remains free on a narrow-based mesentery and is liable to undergo volvulus (Volvulus neonatorum) which if unrecognised is rapidly fatal.

E True Sigmoid volvulus is more common in countries where the diet consists mainly of roughage e.g. Africa.

(For more information, see chs 30 and 31 of Principles and Practice of Surgery)

24. Intestinal surgery

231 Concerning anatomical and physiological characteristics of the intestinal tract:

  A the gut can be divided into three main segments, each with its own principal artery of supply.

  B intestinal pain is mediated by the sympathetic nervous system.

  C the caecum may be situated in the right upper quadrant of the abdomen.

  D the middle third of the rectum lies below the pelvic peritoneal reflection.

  E the descending colon is mainly responsible for active absorption of sodium and water, whilst the ascending colon is a storage organ.

232 The following are true of gastrointestinal surgery:

  A anastomotic leakage is less common following small bowel anastomosis than after large bowel anastomosis.

  B following gastrojejunostomy, anaemia is common.

  C following major resection of the ileum, there is an increased incidence of cholesterol gallstones.

  D following major resection of the small intestine, the resting gastric secretory volume will decrease.

  E the leak rate following colorectal anastomosis, as detected by instillation of a water-soluble contrast medium, is approximately 40%.

(Answers overleaf)

231 A True   The gastrointestinal tract develops from a continuous tube which can be divided into the foregut, midgut and hindgut. Each part of the primitive gut has its own arterial supply (the coeliac axis, the superior mesenteric, and the inferior mesenteric arteries respectively).

B True   The mesentery of the intestine has a rich autonomic (visceral) nerve supply. The sympathetic and parasympathetic nerves influence motility, blood flow and secretion. Intestinal pain is mediated through the sympathetic nervous system.

C True   The most common congenital anomaly of intestinal rotation is failed caecal descent, which means that the caecum may adopt a position in the right upper quadrant.

D False   It is peritonealised anteriorly and laterally in its upper third, and its middle third has a peritoneal covering anteriorly; however, the lower third lies completely below the pelvic peritoneal reflections.

E False   Sodium and water absorption occurs mainly in the right colon; the left side acts as a reservoir prior to defaecation.

232 A True   The small bowel has a more plentiful blood supply, a stronger wall and a luminal content which is liquid and contains very few bacteria.

B True   The duodenum is mainly responsible for absorption of fat and iron, and in the creation of a gastro-jejunostomy chyme will bypass the duodenum and pass into the efferent limb of the gastro-enterostomy.

C True   The loss of water and bile salts results in an imbalance between cholesterol and bile salts in the bile contained in the gallbladder, resulting in a supersaturation of cholesterol and consequently calculus formation.

D False   Following large small-bowel resections, massive gastric hypersecretion is common, possibly due to loss of intestinal inhibitory hormones. Consequently the low luminal pH compounds malabsorption by inactivating intestinal lipase and trypsin. E True The radiological leak rate is significantly higher than those leaks which are clinically significant (5–10%).

(For more information, see ch 29 of Principles and Practice of Surgery)

233 Regarding abdominal stomas:

A it is important to mark the site preoperatively.

B an ileostomy is usually sited in the right iliac fossa and has an everted spout.

C a feeding jejunostomy is frequently employed in multiply traumatised patients, and in malnourished patients undergoing extensive resections for upper gastrointestinal malignancy.

D construction of a loop ileostomy reduces the anastomotic leak rate following low anterior resection of the rectum and restorative proctocolectomy.

E renal and biliary calculi are common in patients with an end colostomy.

234 Concerning intestinal diverticula:

A the congenital Meckel's diverticulum may cause severe gastrointestinal bleeding.

B solitary diverticulum of the caecum is an acquired phenomenon.

C colonic diverticula are mucosal herniations at sites where blood vessels penetrate the muscular coat of the intestinal wall.

D rectal bleeding is a common presenting feature of sigmoid diverticulitis.

E perforated sigmoid diverticular disease is best managed by resection of the diseased segment and primary anastomosis.

(Answers overleaf)

233 A True   This gives the patient the opportunity to wear an appliance on the proposed site for a period of time, and experiment with the position of the stoma so that the best site can be chosen for each individual patient.

B True   The site is not always consistent, especially when complications have occurred necessitating re-siting of the stoma. The presence of a spout is more reliable in recognising an ileostomy.

C True   By commencing enteral feeding early in the postoperative period, it is possible to prevent atrophy of intestinal villi and mucosal barrier breakdown and thus (a) reduce the perioperative morbidity, especially from nosocomial pneumonia, and (b) offset the catabolic response to surgery.

D False   There is no evidence that creating a loop ileostomy or colostomy decreases the rate of anastomotic breakdown in low colorectal anastomoses. The advantage is that should an anastomotic leak occur, the bowel is defunctioned preventing faecal spillage and peritoneal contamination.

E False   There are minimal fluid losses from a colostomy, but considerable losses from an ileostomy. Considerable loss of water from the system increases the incidence of calculus formation.

234 A True   Meckel's diverticulum may become obstructed and present like acute appendicitis; it may also ulcerate, perforate, bleed or undergo malignant transformation, largely as a result of the heterotopic mucosa which is present in 50% of cases. Only 5% of Meckel's diverticula cause symptoms.

B False   This is a rare congenital lesion, which when inflamed will present like acute appendicitis and at operation is frequently indistinguishable from a caecal neoplasm.

C True   Diverticula are due to an abnormality of colonic motility with incoordination of contractility. This causes pain, constipation and herniation of mucosa between the mesenteric and antimesenteric taeniae, where the blood vessels penetrate the circular muscle.

D False   Rectal bleeding from colonic diverticula is well recognised, but is extremely rare compared with the other complications associated with this disease, namely acute inflammation, perforation, pericolic abscess and fistula formation, and obstruction.

E False   Primary anastomosis is not recommended in acute diverticular disease or in any condition where there is a septic focus.

(For more information, see ch 29 of Principles and Practice of Surgery)

235 Crohn's disease:

  A affects the colon in isolation in <10% of patients.

  B is a transmural condition with a propensity for abscess and fistula formation.

  C has submucosal non-caseating granulomata as a characteristic histopathological feature.

  D may result in toxic dilatation of the colon.

  E of the small bowel is best managed by resection of the diseased segments with a margin of healthy intestine.

236 In Crohn's disease:

  A steroids are employed to maintain remission of the disease.

  B sulphasalazine is of limited benefit as maintenance therapy in colonic Crohn's.

  C combination antituberculous therapy frequently results in a decrease in the Crohn's disease activity index (CDAI).

  D <50% of patients require surgical intervention.

  E recrudescence of the disease frequently occurs at the site of previous anastomosis.

(Answers overleaf)

235 A False   There are three broad categories: (1) disease affecting the terminal ileum in isolation (55%); (2) colonic disease in isolation (25%); and (3) panenteric disease (20%).

    B True   The propensity for transmural inflammation and the characteristic appearance of deep fissured 'rose thorn' ulcers predispose to local abscess and fistula formation.

    C True   This is a characteristic of Crohn's disease and is encountered in approximately 50% of specimens. Granulomata also occur in a small number of patients with ulcerative colitis.

    D True   This is more common in ulcerative colitis but may also occur in infective colitis (shigellosis, salmonellosis, enteropathic E. coli, clostridial and campylobacter colitis) and Crohn's disease.

    E False   Resections should be limited where possible, as recurrence is common and should be limited where possible, as recurrence is common and useful nutritional and absorptive surface area is lost if surgery is not conservative. Stricturoplasty provides the best option in short, chronic strictures as it relieves the obstruction while conserving intestine.

236 A False   Steroids and other immunosuppressants, e.g. azathiaprine, have been employed in acute exacerbations but their long-term use is to be avoided.

    B False   Large bowel disease frequently responds well to sulphasalazine, but small bowel disease will not respond, as indigenous colonic flora are required to metabolise the drug to its active compounds, namely sulphapyridine and 5-aminosalicylic acid.

    C True   Combination antituberculous therapy has been shown to be efficacious in a small population of patients with medically refractory Crohn's disease. The basis for this treatment is the implication of an infective aetiology (mycobacteria paratuberculosis).

    D False   Almost 90% of patients with Crohn's disease will require surgery at some stage. The risk of recurrence requiring surgical treatment is approximately 6% per year.

    E True   Theories include: (a) impairment of the blood supply at the anastomosis; and (b) relative stagnation of luminal contents at the site of the anastomosis.

(For more information, see ch 29 of Principles and Practice of Surgery)

237 In ulcerative colitis:

   A patients may present with obstructive jaundice.
   B there is an increased incidence in cigarette smokers.
   C double-contrast barium enema is the investigation of choice in acute colitis.
   D patients developing colonic malignancy have a better prognosis than patients developing sporadic neoplasia de novo.
   E treated by restorative proctocolectomy, those patients developing pouchitis are best treated by local steroid enemata.

238 In intestinal ischaemia:

   A approximately 30% of patients have no evidence of arterial or venous occlusion.
   B patients usually present catastrophically with signs of generalised peritonitis.
   C serum inorganic phosphate is considerably reduced.
   D there is a good response to an infusion of sandostatin.
   E of the colon, there is a predilection for the splenic flexure.

(Answers overleaf)

237 A True   Patients with inflammatory bowel disease due to
either Crohn's disease or ulcerative colitis may
develop sclerosing cholangitis as one of a number
of extra-enteric features of the disease. Others
include arthritis, iritis, and vascular skin rashes
(erythema nodosum, pyoderma gangrenosum).

   B False   This is one condition which has a lower incidence
in smokers.

   C False   It is important to exclude dilatation of the colon
and perforation by plain abdominal and chest
radiography.

   D False   The cancers are flatter and more occult in their
presentation. They may be multifocal and have a
worse prognosis than sporadic colorectal
carcinomata.

   E False   The incidence of clinical pouchitis is 20% and it
responds well to a course of metronidazole in most
cases.

238 A True   Nonocclusive mesenteric infarction is associated
with low cardiac output, which may have an
obvious cause (sepsis, cardiac failure, hypovolaemia) or may be entirely occult.

   B False   This disease is known for its symptoms being out
of keeping with the findings on abdominal
examination ('disease of symptoms not signs').

   C False   Serum inorganic phosphate concentrations are
elevated and, combined with the presence of a
metabolic acidosis on arterial blood gas analysis,
provide a reasonably sensitive test of intestinal
ischaemia.

   D False   Sandostatin is a splanchnic vasoconstrictor which
has no value, and would only compound the
problem of intestinal ischaemia.

   E True   This area has the most tenuous blood supply
marking the watershed between the superior and
inferior mesenteric arterial blood supplies.

(For more information, see ch 29 of Principles and Practice of Surgery)

239 Concerning intestinal polyps:
  A the multiple polyps in the Peutz–Jeghers syndrome are adenomatous in nature.
  B adenomatous polyps are the commonest colonic polyps.
  C colonic villous adenomas may result in hypokalaemia.
  D familial adenomatous polyposis exhibits an autosomal dominant inheritance pattern.
  E familial adenomatous polyposis (FAP) is associated with an increased incidence of other malignant neoplasms.

240 Large bowel carcinoma:
  A is the commonest cause of male cancer deaths.
  B has a propensity for the rectosigmoid region.
  C has a family history in 25% of cases.
  D has an overall 5-year survival of 50%.
  E with liver metastases is incurable.

(Answers overleaf)

239 **A** **False** The polyps seen in this condition are not neoplastic, but are hamartomatous.

    B **False** The commonest colonic polyps are hyperplastic 'metaplastic' polyps. These are small, usually sessile, pale, oval nodules, seldom measuring more than 5 mm in diameter.

    C **True** These polyps are renowned for their ability to secrete potassium-rich mucus resulting in hypokalaemia.

    D **True** This rare autosomal dominant syndrome is caused by an inherited defect in the adenomatous polyposis coli (APC) gene on chromosome 5.

    E **True** There is an increased incidence of desmoid tumours, papillary carcinoma of the thyroid and periampullary carcinoma.

240 **A** **False** Carcinoma of the colon and rectum is second only to lung cancer as a cause of cancer death in the Western world, where there is a higher incidence and a lifetime risk of approximately 1 in 22 for males and 1 in 33 for females.

    B **True** Two-thirds of large bowel carcinomas occur in the rectosigmoid region.

    C **True** The risk of developing a colonic carcinoma rises to 1 in 10 if a first degree relative is affected. Recent interest has centred on a defective gene on chromosome 2 which is implicated in some 15% of cases.

    D **True** Duke A — no spread beyond the muscularis mucosa (10% of patients, ~90% 5-year survival); Duke B — spread through bowel wall to serosa (33% of patients, ~66% 5-year survival); Duke C — spread to involve lymph nodes (33% of patients, ~33% 5-year survival); Duke D — distant metastases (33% of patients, ~0–5% 5-year survival).

    E **False** 5–10% of patients are suitable for curative resection. Provided the number of metastases is <3 and these are isolated to one lobe of the liver with no evidence of extrahepatic disease, patients may undergo hepatic resection and some centres have demonstrated a 30% 5-year survival rate in this patient population.

(For more information, see ch 29 of Principles and Practice of Surgery)

25. Anorectal conditions

241 Concerning the anal canal:

  A it is 3–4 cm in length and is lined with columnar epithelium.
  B it has two sphincters, both of which are under autonomic control.
  C it has an internal sphincter which is the major determinant of faecal continence.
  D it receives its blood supply solely from branches of the internal iliac artery.
  E its lymphatic drainage is to the superficial inguinal glands.

242 Anal continence is dependent upon:

  A the ability to appreciate anal distension.
  B secretion of bombesin.
  C intact anal sensation.
  D normal pudendal nerve function.
  E normal anal cushions.

(Answers overleaf)

241 A False   The lower two thirds of the anal canal are lined
               with stratified squamous epithelium, and the upper
               third with columnar epithelium.

   B False   The internal sphincter is under strictly involuntary
               (autonomic) control; the external sphincter is
               striated muscle supplied by somatic branches from
               the pudendal nerve.

   C True   The internal sphincter contributes as much as 80%
               of the resting pressure within the anal canal, the
               remaining 20% coming from the external sphincter.

   D False   The superior rectal artery is a continuation of the
               inferior mesenteric artery and forms three branches
               (two right and one left) which descend the rectum
               to supply the anal canal.

   E True   Inflammatory and neoplastic diseases of the anus
               drain to the internal iliac nodes and to the
               superficial inguinal nodes.

242 A False   The main determinant is the ability of the rectum to
               appreciate distension. Once the rectum is full, the
               internal sphincter relaxes and the external sphincter
               maintains continence.

   B False
   C True   The receptors in the anal mucosa permit subtle
               discrimination between flatus and faeces.

   D True   The pudendal nerve supplies the external sphincter.
               This can be objectively assessed by means of
               electromyography which can map a deficient
               sphincter and determine the degree of pudendal
               nerve latency.

   E False   The anal cushions may contribute to closure of the
               anal canal through their physical bulk, but they
               certainly cannot be considered a major determinant
               in anal continence.

(For more information, see ch 32 of Principles and Practice of Surgery)

243 The following conditions can result in faecal incontinence:

A ulcerative colitis.
B rectal prolapse.
C diabetes mellitus.
D chordoma.
E benign intracranial hypertension.

244 Haemorrhoids:

A are venous varicosities in the anal canal.
B have an arterial component.
C are an acquired phenomenon.
D which prolapse beyond the anal verge but reduce spontaneously are second degree.
E when prolapsed and thrombosed are painful and should be treated by urgent haemorrhoidectomy.

(Answers overleaf)

243 A True Severe diarrhoea can occasionally result in incontinence by overwhelming the sphincter with a high volume of watery stool.

B True Complete rectal prolapse is often associated with incontinence, possibly due to both perineal descent and damage to the internal anal sphincter from repeated dilation of the anus by the prolapse.

C True Diabetes frequently results in autonomic neuropathy which affects the involuntary control of the internal sphincter.

D True Neurological disease affecting the innervation of the sphincters (S2–S4) and anal mucosa occasionally leads to incontinence, e.g. tumours or trauma to the sacral cord and cauda equina as well as demyelinating disease.

E True Cerebrovascular disease and the dementias commonly result in incontinence, particularly if the patient develops faecal impaction.

244 A False The anal lining is formed into roughly separate pads composed of a sponge-like venous plexus supported by elastic tissue and smooth muscle. The anal submucosal muscle (muscularis submucosae ani) acts to prevent the anal cushions being dragged downwards and out with the stool. Piles result as a failure of this mechanism.

B True Arterioles are numerous and can be traced directly into the saccules.

C False These discrete venous dilatations are found at birth and characterise the veins of the haemorrhoidal venous plexus in the submucosa of the anal lining, both above and below the dentate line.

D True Internal piles are graded in four degrees: first degree bulge into the anal canal but do not prolapse; second degree prolapse through the anus but return spontaneously; third degree remain prolapsed, requiring digital reduction; and fourth degree prolapse chronically and cannot be returned to the anal canal.

E False Because of the severe degree of oedema and inflammatory response, it is unwise to operate urgently on prolapsed thrombosed piles as this frequently will compromise the normal anal mucosa and may predispose to anal stenosis.

(For more information, see ch 32 of Principles and Practice of Surgery)·

245 Internal haemorrhoids:

   A are palpable on rectal examination.
   B arise above the dentate line.
   C respond well to medical therapy.
   D may be treated by injection of 50% phenol.
   E treated by haemorrhoidectomy are commonly complicated by secondary haemorrhage.

246 Rectal prolapse:

   A has a male preponderance.
   B is strictly a disease of adulthood.
   C commonly occurs in morbidly obese patients.
   D may result in the solitary rectal ulcer syndrome.
   E repair may result in constipation and/or incontinence.

247 Primary fissure-in-ano:

   A frequently presents with painless rectal bleeding.
   B is situated posteriorly in >80% of cases.
   C may be suspected by the presence of a hypertrophied skin tag on inspection of the anus.
   D is commonly a self-limiting condition with a high rate of spontaneous healing.
   E may be treated effectively by division of the internal anal sphincter.

(Answers overleaf)

245 **A** **False**   Proctoscopy is the main tool for demonstrating internal piles.

B **True**   Internal infers that the piles arise above the dentate line.

C **False**   Cream and suppositories are usually inadequate, offering little benefit to the patient.

D **False**   The phenol used in injection of piles is 10% phenol in almond oil. Use of a higher concentration of phenol may cause irreparable damage to the anal complex.

E **False**   Although this is a well recognised complication, its frequency is less than 1%. Reactionary haemorrhage occurs in 2% of individuals.

246 **A** **False**   Approximately 85% of affected adults are women, and elderly women are particularly at risk.

B **False**   Rectal prolapse can occur in childhood and is usually a partial or mucosal prolapse.

C **False**   It is more likely to occur in malnourished individuals.

D **True**   The pathophysiology is due to recurrent prolapse of the anterior rectal wall and is demonstrable by defaecating proctography.

E **True**   Incontinence occurs in around 30% of patients following rectopexy, as a result of recurrent prolapse of the rectum through the sphincter mechanism. A similar proportion of patients experience constipation, due to the rigid fixation of the rectum compounded by disturbance of the sacral plexus following excessive rectal mobilisation.

247 **A** **False**   This is usually an extremely painful condition.

B **True**   In 15% of females and 1% of males, primary anal fissures occur anteriorly. Secondary fissures are less consistent in their site and may be multiple.

C **True**   Inflammation around the fissure results in swelling of the margins of the fissure, and an oedematous skin tag develops at the anal verge. This is known as a 'sentinel pile'.

D **False**   Spontaneous healing is uncommon because the spasm of the anal sphincter prevents proper drainage of the chronically contaminated fissure.

E **True**   Two main treatment strategies are currently employed; (1) anal dilatation; (2) formal division of the internal sphincter as either an open or subcutaneous procedure.

(For more information, see ch 32 of Principles and Practice of Surgery)

248 Anorectal abscesses:

A arise following infection in the intersphincteric anal glands.
B of the intersphincteric type usually present less acutely than an ischiorectal abscess.
C may predispose to fissure-in-ano formation.
D when associated with a fistula-in-ano, should have the fistula treated at the time of initial incision and drainage of the abscess.
E upon incision and drainage, should have skin and contents analysed histologically and microbiologically, respectively.

249 A pilonidal nus:

A is a condition exclusive to the natal cleft.
B is not usually symptomatic unless secondarily infected.
C if infected, is effectively treated by simple incision and drainage.
D recurs in approximately 20% of individuals.
E has potential for malignant transformation.

(Answers overleaf)

248 A True   Anal glands situated within the anal crypts are usually the primary site of infection.

   B False   When the abscess is confined to the intersphincteric space there are frequently no external features, although the pain is intense. Rectal examination may reveal induration in the rectal wall. Ischiorectal abscess formation may be more indolent as this is a capacious space filled with loose fat lobules. It can become extensive and track around the rectum posteriorly, forming a 'horseshoe abscess'.

   C False   Abscess which points into the bowel lumen and through the perianal skin simultaneously or which is incised externally may result in fistula-in-ano formation.

   D False   A fistula will not be immediately apparent; 10 days after incision and drainage a further examination of the rectum and anus should be carried out under anaesthetic to confirm or exclude the presence of a fistula.

   E True   Histology of the abscess may reveal granulomata suggesting Crohn's disease. If enteric bacteria are isolated then fistula is likely.

249 A False   Although this is the commonest site, they are occasionally seen in old surgical wounds (particularly in the perineum), in the interdigital clefts of barbers and taxidermists, and in the anal sphincter muscle.

   B False   It may be asymptomatic but usually presents with local discomfort, discharge and acute abscess formation, which is frequently recurrent.

   C False   Incision and drainage of a pilonidal abscess is effective only in relieving the pain and the acute septic insult. There is a 50% recurrence rate after simple incision and drainage.

   D True   Many surgical strategies are described for dealing with pilonidal sinus and abscess, which reflects that none are particularly successful.

   E True   As with any chronically infected sinus, a Marjolin's ulcer can arise.

(For more information, see ch 32 of Principles and Practice of Surgery)

250 In anal cancer:

   A >80% of cases are squamous cell in origin.
   B basal cell carcinoma and melanoma constitute a small
         proportion of cases.
   C surgical resection is the first-line the therapy.
   D occult metastasis to superficial inguinal lymph nodes is
         common.
   E there is an association with a sexually transmissible agent.

(Answers overleaf)

250 **A** **True**
    B **True** Other primary anal malignancies include malignant melanoma, adenocarcinoma, malignant lymphoma and basal carcinoma.
    C **False** There has been a move away from radical surgery as the primary treatment for anal squamous carcinoma is radiotherapy.
    D **False** Only 15% of patients will have involved superficial inguinal nodes at presentation and a further 10% will develop lymphadenopathy during the course of their illness.
    E **True** It has been suggested that the human papilloma virus (HPV) might be important in the development of anal cancer.

(For more information, see ch 32 of Principles and Practice of Surgery)

26. The liver and biliary tract

251 Appropriate radiological investigations of the liver and biliary tract include:

A ultrasonography.
B intravenous cholangiogram in a patient with obstructive jaundice.
C oral cholecystogram in a patient with obstructive jaundice.
D CT scan in a patient with obstructive jaundice.
E nuclear magnetic resonance (MRI) scan.

252 The following statements are true:

A in haemolytic jaundice there are high circulating levels of conjugated bilirubin and no bilirubin in the urine.
B in obstructive jaundice there are high circulating levels of conjugated bilirubin and bilirubin in the urine.
C in obstructive jaundice there is excess urobilinogen in the urine which renders it dark in colour.
D in obstructive jaundice the serum alkaline phosphatase rises.
E in hepatocellular jaundice there is no rise in the serum alkaline phosphatase.

253 Clinical stigmata of chronic liver disease include:

A spider naevi.
B koilonychia.
C finger clubbing.
D caput Medusa.
E peripheral oedema.

(Answers overleaf)

251 A True   This will detect gallstones, biliary dilatation and space-occupying lesions in the liver and pancreas.

B False   Contrast in the venous system must be conjugated to bilirubin and excreted in the bile, to outline the biliary system. In obstructive jaundice, excretion into the biliary system cannot occur.

C False   For the same reason as in **B**— in a patient with obstructive jaundice the appropriate cholangiographic investigations are PTC and ERCP.

D True   This can be used to identify hepatic, bile duct and pancreatic tumours.

E True   This is very accurate for some specific lesions of the liver (e.g. a haemangioma, which produces a classical appearance following intravenous contrast enhancement).

252 A False   There are high serum levels of unconjugated bilirubin and no bilirubin in the urine.

B True   Conjugated bilirubin is water-soluble and is excreted in the urine.

C False   Urobilinogen is absent from the urine.

D True   Due to increased formation in the cells lining the biliary canaliculi. The rise in serum alkaline phosphatase precedes the rise in bilirubin and its fall is more gradual once obstruction is relieved.

E False   Oedema of the hepatic parenchyma in hepato-cellular jaundice produces slight intrahepatic biliary obstruction and a modest rise in the serum alkaline phosphatase.

253 A True   These are due to high oestrogen concentration and are found in the drainage area of the superior vena cava.

B False   This occurs in iron deficiency anaemia. In chronic liver disease, leuconychia (white nails) may occur in association with hypoproteinaemia.

C True

D True   This refers to dilatation of abdominal wall veins radiating from the umbilicus, which may occur in portal hypertension.

E True   Due to hypoproteinaemia and secondary hyperaldosteronism.

(For more information, see ch 33 of Principles and Practice of Surgery)

254 In chronic liver disease:

    A transaminase enzyme levels >1000 IU indicate
        that the patient is classified as Child–Pugh grade C.

    B portal hypertension may result in oesophageal variceal
        bleeding.

    C portal hypertension may result in haemorrhoid
        development.

    D a fine tremor classically occurs in an encephalopathic
        patient.

    E encephalopathy may be precipitated by an oesophageal
        variceal bleed.

**255 Concerning the management of bleeding oesophageal
varices:**

    A all patients with known oesophageal varices who present
        with profuse haematemesis should have a Sengstaken tube
        inserted.

    B pharmacological therapy commonly used involves
        intravenous somatosatin.

    C injection sclerotherapy cannot be used in an acutely
        bleeding patient.

    D the majority of patients will require insertion of a
        Sengstaken tube.

    E a Sengstaken-Blakemore tube has three lumens.

**256 The following conditions predispose to gallstone
formation:**

    A giardiasis.

    B cirrhosis.

    C diabetes mellitus.

    D choledochal cyst.

    E infestation of the biliary tract with *Clonorchis sinensis*.

(Answers overleaf)

254 A False   The transaminase enzymes are not used in this classification. It uses two biochemical parameters (serum bilirubin and albumin), two clinical parameters (encephalopathy and ascites), and one haematological parameter (prothrombin time).

B True   In the area of portal (left gastric vein)–systemic (azygous vein) anastomosis.

C False   Very rarely, portal hypertension can lead to the development of rectal varices but not haemorrhoids.

D False   The tremor is a coarse 'liver flap' (asterixis).

E True   Due to the large protein load entering the bowel. Treatment with neomycin and lactulose is indicated.

255 A False   Even in patients with known oesophageal varices, haematemesis will be due to a non-variceal cause (e.g. peptic ulcer) in approximately 30%.

B False   But octreotide, an eight-amino acid analogue of somatostatin, is commonly used as it is much less expensive.

C False

D False   This is rarely required; in most cases, bleeding will stop following the use of pharmacological methods or injection sclerotherapy.

E False   It has four — one to inflate the gastric balloon, one to inflate the oesophageal balloon, one to aspirate the pharynx and oesophagus, and one to aspirate the stomach. Great care must be taken when inserting the tube as, if it is not correctly positioned in the stomach, inflation of the gastric balloon can result in rupture of the oesophagus.

256 A False
B True
C True
D True   In this condition, cystic dilatation of the biliary tract results in bile stasis, recurrent cholangitis and an increased risk of gallstone formation.

E True

(For more information, see ch 33 of Principles and Practice of Surgery)

257 The following statements are true:

A   a stone impacted in the common hepatic duct will produce a mucocele of the gallbladder.

B   a stone impacted at Hartmann's pouch will usually produce obstructive jaundice.

C   biliary obstruction due to stones often leads to secondary infection.

D   recurrent obstruction and infection due to stone disease may ultimately lead to primary biliary cirrhosis.

E   gallstones occur more frequently in patients with Crohn's disease.

258 Concerning tumours of the biliary tract:

A   gallstones predispose to carcinoma of the gallbladder.

B   a choledochal cyst predisposes to cholangiocarcinoma.

C   cholangiocarcinoma can occur as a multifocal condition affecting the intrahepatic biliary tree.

D   cholangiocarcinoma rarely involves the bile duct confluence (junction of right and left hepatic ducts).

E   cholangiocarcinoma tends to metastasise widely.

259 The following statements are true:

A   sclerosing cholangitis has an increased incidence in patients with inflammatory bowel disease.

B   hepatocellular carcinoma may be associated with increased serum human chorionic gonadotrophin (HCG) concentration.

C   hepatic adenomas occur most frequently in males.

D   in the Budd–Chiari syndrome there is primary thrombosis and obstruction of the portal vein.

E   the presence of multiple cysts arising within the liver parenchyma is known as Caroli's disease.

(Answers overleaf)

257 A False   This is caused by impaction of a stone in Hartmann's pouch or cystic duct; if a mucocele becomes infected, an empyema results.

B False   The common hepatic and common bile ducts remain patent. One very rare exception is when gross inflammation around a stone in Hartmann's pouch also involves the common bile duct and produces jaundice (Mirizzi syndrome).

C True   Known as cholangitis; this results in jaundice, pain and rigors (Charcot's triad).

D False   It may lead to secondary biliary cirrhosis. Primary biliary cirrhosis is an autoimmune condition, characteristically affecting middle-aged females and associated with antimitochondrial antibodies in the serum.

E True   Due to disruption of the enterohepatic recirculation of bile salts.

258 A True

B True   Due to chronic bile stasis, recurrent cholangitis and stone formation.

C True

D False   It frequently occurs here (known in this site as a Klatskin tumour).

E False   Although this is an aggressive tumour associated with a poor prognosis, widespread systemic metastasis is not usually a feature.

259 A True   This is a condition characterised by areas of fibrous stricturing in the intra- and extrahepatic biliary systems. It typically occurs in males and, if extensive, may lead to secondary biliary cirrhosis and liver failure.

B False   It may be associated with an increased serum alphafetoprotein concentration.

C False   They are rare tumours, which occur almost exclusively in females and may be causally related to the oral contraceptive pill.

D False   The primary problem involves thrombosis and obstruction of the hepatic veins. Secondary portal hypertension may develop.

E False   This is polycystic liver disease, which may occur in association with polycystic kidneys. Caroli's disease is characterised by congenital cystic dilatation of the intrahepatic bile ducts.

(For more information, see ch 33 of Principles and Practice of Surgery)

260 The following statements are true:

A oral bile salt therapy for 3 months is an effective way to dissolve gallstones.

B in order to remove common bile duct (CBD) stones (choledocholithiasis), surgical exploration of the CBD is necessary.

C gallstone ileus occurs following passage of a stone through the sphincter of Oddi into the gastrointestinal tract.

D if a T-tube cholangiogram reveals retained CBD stones, these may be removed via the T-tube tract.

E a cholecystectomy should always be performed in a young patient in whom gallstones are discovered incidentally (e.g. during ultrasound scanning in pregnancy).

(Answers overleaf)

260 **A False**   Treatment is required for up to 2 years. After
discontinuation of therapy, stones will recur; in
addition, the primary problem (the presence of the
diseased gallbladder) has not been removed.

   B False   This may also be performed by ERCP and
sphincterotomy, and in elderly, frail patients this
may be the preferred method.

   C False   In order to cause obstruction of the gastrointestinal
tract a large stone must pass via a fistula between
the gallbladder and duodenum (cholecyst–duodenal
fistula). The classic appearance on a plain
abdominal film is that of signs of small bowel
obstruction (air/fluid levels), an image of the stone
and air in the biliary tree.

   D True   This is known as a Burhenne procedure.

   E False   A large Scandinavian study has shown that the
incidence of future gallbladder disease in these
patients is no higher than in the general
population.

(For more information, see ch 33 of Principles and Practice of Surgery)

27. The pancreas

The spleen

261 **Causes of acute pancreatitis include:**
- **A** gallstones.
- **B** alcohol abuse.
- **C** hypocalcaemia.
- **D** hyperlipidaemia.
- **E** spironolactone.

262 **The following parameters indicate the presence of severe disease in patients with acute pancreatitis:**
- **A** serum amylase >1000 IU.
- **B** blood glucose <10 mmol/l.
- **C** white cell count >15 × 10^9/l.
- **D** total bilirubin >55 μmol/l.
- **E** serum lactate dehydrogenase (LDH) >350 μmol/l.

263 **The following are recognised complications of acute pancreatitis:**
- **A** haemorrhagic necrosis.
- **B** renal failure.
- **C** pseudocyst.
- **D** hypercalcaemia.
- **E** abscess formation.

(Answers overleaf)

261 **A** **True**   Approximately 40–50% of cases are associated with gallstones.

      B **True**   The proportion of cases linked to alcohol varies around the world: in Scotland it is approximately 30%, while in France and North America it is as high as 60–90%.

      C **False**   Hypercalcaemia.

      D **True**

      E **False**   But some drugs are associated with pancreatitis (e.g. thiazide diuretics and steroids).

262 **A** **False**   A serum amylase above this level is used to diagnose acute pancreatitis — it is not a severity criterion.

      B **False**   In severe acute pancreatitis the serum glucose would rise due to tissue destruction and compromise of endocrine function.

      C **True**

      D **False**   This is not used as a severity criterion.

      E **True**   The above answers are based on the Imrie prognostic criteria for acute pancreatitis; there are eight criteria, and the presence of three or more signifies severe disease). The Ranson system is fairly similar.

263 **A** **True**   If severe, this results in leakage of pancreatic enzymes and blood into the abdominal cavity, with bruising around the umbilicus (Cullen's sign) and in the flanks (Grey–Turner's sign).

      B **True**   Remote organ failure (e.g. renal failure, respiratory failure) may occur secondary to the acute inflammatory reaction with release of cytokines and other inflammatory mediators.

      C **True**   This is a collection of fluid within the lesser sac enclosed within a thick granulation membrane. It may bleed or perforate, and if it does not resolve spontaneously, internal drainage into the stomach (cystogastrostomy) may be necessary.

      D **False**   Hypocalcaemia occurs.

      E **True**   Surgical drainage may be necessary. In severe cases, the abdomen may be left open into the lesser sac to allow daily lavage and further drainage of necrotic/infected pancreatic tissue (laparostomy plus necrosectomy).

(For more information, see chs 34 and 35 of Principles and Practice of Surgery)

264   Concerning treatment of acute pancreatitis:

  A conservative management (nil orally, intravenous fluids and nasogastric suction) is sufficient in the vast majority of cases.

  B octreotide is of proven therapeutic benefit.

  C in gallstone pancreatitis, cholecystectomy should be performed 6–8 weeks after the acute attack has resolved.

  D gallstone pancreatitis may be treated by ERCP and sphincterotomy.

  E broad-spectrum antibiotics should be used routinely.

265   Carcinoma of the pancreas:

  A is increasing in incidence in the Western world.

  B is resectable in approximately 50% of cases.

  C may present with an epigastric mass which moves with respiration.

  D is associated with thrombophlebitis migrans.

  E is more common in maturity onset diabetics.

266   The following statements are true:

  A patients with endocrine tumours of the pancreas may have associated tumours of the parathyroid glands and anterior pituitary.

  B insulinomas are usually malignant.

  C glucagonoma is usually associated with diarrhoea, hypokalaemia and achlorhydria.

  D carcinoma of the ampulla of Vater is associated with a better prognosis than pancreatic cancer.

  E glucagonoma is associated with necrotising dermatitis, stomatitis, glossitis, diarrhoea and anaemia.

267   Causes of splenomegaly include:

  A myelofibrosis.

  B chronic myeloid leukaemia.

  C coeliac disease.

  D thyrotoxicosis.

  E idiopathic thrombocytopenic purpura (ITP).

(Answers overleaf)

264 A True
   B False   Theoretically, octreotide, by reducing upper gastrointestinal and pancreatic secretion, should be of therapeutic benefit, but this has not been substantiated in clinical trials.
   C False   There is a significant risk of a recurrent attack within this time. Cholecystectomy and operative cholangiography should be performed during the acute hospital admission (3–6 days after the acute attack).
   D True   Particularly in older patients in whom there is a significant operative risk associated with cholecystectomy.
   E False   Pancreatitis is not due to bacterial infection. Antibiotics may be indicated if secondary bacterial infection and abscess formation occur.

265 A True
   B False   It is resectable in less than 10% of cases, usually due to local invasion of the portal or superior mesenteric vein or distant metastases.
   C False   The pancreas is a fixed retroperitoneal organ.
   D True
   E True

266 A True   Multiple endocrine neoplasia (MEN) type 1.
   B False   90% are benign and solitary.
   C False   This is true of the VIPoma, a rare benign tumour of the pancreas which secretes vasoactive intestinal peptide (VIP). The syndrome is known as 'pancreatic cholera' or Verner–Morrison syndrome.
   D True   Although it generally presents in the same way, this tumour is much smaller and slower growing. Hence it is important to distinguish it from pancreatic cancer.
   E True   As with the VIPoma, the gastrointestinal symptoms may be controlled by octreotide.

267 A True   In this, the spleen is grossly enlarged.
   B True   Also causes gross splenomegaly.
   C False   In this, the spleen may atrophy.
   D False   This may be associated with splenic atrophy.
   E True   Although the spleen is palpably enlarged in only 2–3% of cases.

(For more information, see chs 34 and 35 of Principles and Practice of Surgery)

268 Primary indications for splenectomy include:

   A hereditary spherocytosis.
   B portal hypertension.
   C Hodgkin's disease.
   D trauma.
   E Felty's syndrome.

269 Effects of splenectomy include:

   A leucopenia.
   B thrombocytosis.
   C increased numbers of abnormal haematological cell types.
   D increased serum IgM levels.
   E impaired phagocytosis.

270 Recommended therapeutic measures to counteract the effects of splenectomy include:

   A treatment with warfarin to counteract an increased risk of venous thrombosis due to thrombocytosis.
   B administration of pneumococcal vaccine.
   C venesection.
   D long-term antibiotic therapy.
   E administration of influenza vaccine.

(Answers overleaf)

268 A True Gallstones may also be present and cholecystectomy should be carried out simultaneously.

B False Portal hypertension per se is not an indication for
splenectomy; however, splenectomy may be
performed as part of a surgical procedure to reduce
portal pressure (e.g. distal spleno-renal shunt
(Warren shunt).

C True

D True Although in recent years increasing attempts are
being made to salvage the spleen, e.g. suture or
mesh repair (splenorrhaphy).

E True Splenomegaly occurs in association with chronic
rheumatoid arthritis. There is a neutropenia which
renders patients more susceptible to infection and
which is usually reversed by splenectomy. The
arthritis is unaffected by splenectomy.

269 A False There is leucocytosis, maximal 7–10 days after
splenectomy.

B True Again, maximal 7–10 days after splenectomy; the
thrombocytosis may persist for many years.

C True Manifested by Howell–Jolly bodies and target cells.

D False The serum IgM falls initially but normalises with
time. The IgG and IgA level remains constant.

E True Due to several factors, including a prolonged fall in
plasma tuftsin levels and impaired complement
activation via the alternative pathway.

270 A False Full anticoagulation is not necessary, but prophylactic heparin should be given in the perioperative
period. If thrombocytosis persists aspirin therapy is
indicated.

B True Following splenectomy there is an increased
incidence of infection with pneumococci and other
encapsulated organisms. Pneumococcal vaccine
should be given immediately after emergency
splenectomy, and 1–2 months prior to elective
splenectomy. Vaccination is now also given against
Haemophilus influenzae and meningococcus.

C False Not indicated.

D True Usually with penicillin — to counteract the risk of
infection and severe sepsis, known as overwhelm-
ing post splenectomy infection (OPSI). There is
debate over how long antibiotics should be continued — 2 years, 5 years, or lifelong?

E False

(For more information, see chs 34 and 35 of Principles and Practice of Surgery)

28. Urological surgery

271 Concerning urological investigations:

  A proteinuria of >150 mg/24 h suggests an underlying glomerular abnormality.

  B creatinine clearance accurately reflects the glomerular filtration rate and is calculated from the volume of urine passed in 24 hours multipled by the urinary creatinine concentration divided by the plasma creatinine concentration.

  C intravenous urography is an accurate investigation for renal function.

  D nuclear scanning of the kidneys and micturating cystography are the gold standard investigations employed in vesico-ureteric reflux.

  E renal angiography is the investigation of choice in renal carcinoma.

272 Urinary retention:

  A is invariably associated with suprapubic pain.

  B may occur in patients with normal transurethral endoscopic findings.

  C occurring in young females is usually not associated with any significant underlying pathology.

  D may result in renal dysfunction.

  E due to urethral stricture is best managed by insertion of a transurethral catheter.

(Answers overleaf)

271 A True   Proteinuria of this degree is pathological and is
one feature of the nephrotic syndrome. The other
components are hypoalbuminaemia, oedema and
secondary hypercholesterolaemia.

B True   Creatinine clearance accurately reflects renal
function. The formula

$$\frac{\text{urinary creatinine} \times \text{volume of urine}/24\,h}{\text{plasma creatinine}}$$

calculates the creatinine clearance in ml/min
(normal range: 50–120 ml/min).

C False   This is a crude test of renal function. It is the most
commonly used test for assessing anatomy of the
urinary tract.

D True   A micturating cystogram is the gold standard
diagnostic test in this congenital condition. A
dimercaptosuccinic acid (DMSA) scan reveals the
degree of renal parenchymal scarring and gives
accurate differential renal function (%).

E False   This investigation is invasive and outdated. It has
been replaced by ultrasonography, which is
harmless to the patient and allows evaluation
of renal vein involvement and regional
lymphadenopathy.

272 A False   Chronic retention is painless and is usually
associated with overflow incontinence.

B True   Urinary retention may occur with normal urethral
and bladder anatomy. This is indicative of a
functional problem (detrusor–bladder neck
dyssynergia, detrusor–sphincter dyssynergia).

C False   The commonest cause of urinary retention in a
young female is multiple sclerosis.

D True   Post-obstructive uropathy may ensue, particularly if
the retention is chronic. It is usually reversible upon
relief of the obstruction.

E False   Transurethral catheterisation is frequently
impossible. The best way of relieving the retention
is by insertion of a suprapubic catheter.

(For more information, see ch 36 of Principles and Practice of Surgery)

273 Benign nodular hyperplasia of the prostate:
  A most commonly presents with the classical triad of hesitancy, poor stream and post-mictural dribbling.
  B occurs as the result of formation of a large adenoma in the periurethral tissue, as opposed to diffuse prostatic hyperplasia.
  C is always confirmed by digital rectal examination.
  D does not give rise to haematuria.
  E treated by transurethral resection (TURP) results in sterility.

274 Urethral obstruction:
  A when congenital, has a poor prognosis.
  B following major trauma where the pelvis is fractured should be treated by transurethral catheterisation.
  C occurs following para-urethral gland infection in females.
  D is a complication of long-term catheterisation.
  E is the main presenting feature in hypospadias.

275 Ureteric calculi:
  A are visible on plain X-ray in >80% of cases.
  B are common in hypoparathyroidism.
  C cause ureteric colic which responds rapidly to parenterally administered diclofenac.
  D may present with testicular pain.
  E pass spontaneously in 90% of cases.

(Answers overleaf)

273 A True

B True   The adenoma compresses normal prostate tissue to the periphery of the gland forming a pseudocapsule inside the true capsule.

C False   Significant bladder outlet obstruction can occur in the presence of a normal rectal examination, when the only lobe to be enlarged is the middle lobe (not accessible to the examining finger).

D False   This is a relatively common symptom where, with straining, frank haematuria occurs at the end of the stream classically from small veins in the periprostatic plexus.

E True   TURP involves resection of the enlarged prostatic lobes and also the internal sphincter, which results in retrograde ejaculation.

274 A True   Posterior urethral valves are easily treated; however, it is the severe obstructive uropathy and thwarted renal development which compromises the future of the infant.

B False   Transurethral catheterisation should only be attempted after gentle urethrography has excluded a urethral tear; these are frequently partial initially but are converted into a full tear by injudicious catheterisation.

C True   Infection and chronic inflammation in these glands results in urethral narrowing and consequently recurrent infective and obstructive symptoms.

D True   This is one form of iatrogenic stricture. It classically occurs at the penoscrotal junction and is thought to be due to mucosal pressure necrosis.

E False   Occasionally meatal stenosis occurs but the commonest reason for presentation is for aesthetic correction.

275 A True   Over 80% of ureteric and renal calculi in the UK are mixed calcium oxalate/phosphate stones. 10% are magnesium ammonium phosphate with variable amounts of calcium, and the remainder are uric acid stones.

B False   Seen in hyperparathyroidism, where excess calcium and phosphate are excreted in the urine.

C True   This is virtually pathognomonic of ureteric colic. Diclofenac decreases renal blood flow and has an antidiuretic effect which usually affords rapid analgesia in ureteric colic.

D True   In ureteric colic it is common for patients to complain of testicular pain; this is referred pain.

E True   Stones <0.5 cm will normally pass spontaneously.

(For more information, see ch 36 of Principles and Practice of Surgery)

276 Transitional cell tumours:

  A of the kidney are best treated by nephrectomy.
  B are increasing in incidence.
  C of the bladder are usually treatable by transurethral resection.
  D classically present with painless haematuria.
  E do not respond to chemoradiotherapy.

277 Carcinoma of the prostate:

  A is the second commonest cause of cancer death in males.
  B is impalpable rectally in 10–15% of cases.
  C usually presents at an early stage.
  D if confined to the prostate gland is suitable for radical surgery.
  E frequently causes lytic bony metastases.

278 Renal carcinoma:

  A is more common in females.
  B arises in the glomeruli.
  C may present with a pathological fracture.
  D responds well to systemic chemotherapy.
  E is associated with cerebellar haemangioblastoma.

(Answers overleaf)

276 A False This tumour tends to be multifocal and if the kidney is removed in isolation the incidence of recurrence in the remaining ureter is 15–25%; it is therefore necessary to remove the kidney and ipsilateral ureter.

B True The increasing incidence is most probably related to the increase in environmental carcinogens.

C True Transurethral resection of the bladder tumour combined with bimanual examination under anaesthetic forms the mainstay of initial treatment and staging.

D True 80% present with haematuria.

E False When involving the bladder, both intravesical chemotherapy and external radiotherapy are useful strategies.

277 A True It is also the third most common malignancy in males, with 10 000 new cases each year in the UK.

B True The diagnosis should never be made on clinical grounds alone.

C False The nature of the disease is for a nodule of prostatic cancer to commence in the peripheral part of the gland, thus it can grow to a large size before becoming symptomatic.

D True The disease tends to present late and to occur in elderly men with a high incidence of concomitant medical disease which precludes radical surgery. Nevertheless, radical prostatectomy with internal iliac lymph node dissection is feasible.

E False Bony metastases are usually sclerotic and confined to the axial skeleton.

278 A False It is three times more common in males.

B False The tumour arises from the renal tubules.

C True It has a natural propensity for haematogenous spread to bone. Long bones are commonly involved and the nature of the secondary tumour is to be lytic, hence pathological fractures are not uncommon.

D False Surgery forms the mainstay of treatment, with local radiotherapy for para-aortic node metastases. Actinomycin D and immunotherapy have been employed with limited success.

E True A feature of the von Hippel–Lindau syndrome; as is retinoblastoma.

(For more information, see ch 36 of Principles and Practice of Surgery)

279 Concerning genitourinary trauma:
  A blunt trauma resulting in a renal parenchymal laceration requires early surgical exploration.
  B the presence and degree of haematuria reliably reflects the gravity of the urological injury.
  C ureteric damage is most commonly iatrogenic.
  D large testicular haematocoeles are best managed conservatively.
  E in blunt urethral disruption immediate repair is contraindicated.

280 Concerning testicular tumours:
  A teratoma occurs in a younger age group than seminoma.
  B serum alphafetoprotein and β-human chorionic gonadotrophin concentrations are abnormal in 75% of cases of teratomas.
  C carcinoma-in-situ occurs in the contralateral testis in 5% of patients undergoing orchidectomy for a germ cell tumour.
  D seminoma is not radiosensitive.
  E prognosis following chemotherapy for malignant teratoma depends on the extent of the disease at presentation.

(Answers overleaf)

279 A False   Provided there is evidence of a functioning kidney on IVU, and no haemodynamic instability on account of a disrupted kidney, a conservative approach is to be recommended.

B False   Have a high index of suspicion and low threshold for intravenous urography.

C True   The ureter is a retroperitoneal structure which is rarely damaged. It accounts for 3% of all genitourinary injuries. Surgical damage accounts for the majority of injuries, especially in the lower third where it is vulnerable on account of its relative fixity and poor blood supply.

D False   Expanding haematocoeles may threaten the viability of the testis. They should be explored urgently, the haematoma evacuated and tunica albuginea repaired.

E False   Exploring acutely with fresh haematoma increases the risk of infection and haemorrhage; however, it is described by. Most would manage this conservatively initially with suprapubic bladder drainage.

280 A True   The peak incidence for teratoma and seminoma occurs between the ages of 20–35 and 25–40 years, respectively.

B True   Tumour markers are useful: (a) as a diagnostic aid, (b) in staging, (c) in determining progonsis, (d) for assessing response to treatment, (e) for detecting relapse and (f) potentially for immunolocalisation.

C True   Approximately 50% will progress to frank malignancy within 5 years. Carcinoma-in-situ is extremely sensitive to low-dose radiotherapy.

D False   This is one of the most radiosensitive human malignancies. It is used in stage I seminoma both locally and prophylactically to para-aortic lymph nodes.

E True   This is the single most important parameter, therefore early diagnosis is essential.

(For more information, see ch 36 of Principles and Practice of Surgery)

29. Neurosurgery

281 Increased intracranial pressure, if unrelieved, may typically be associated with:
A tachycardia.
B hypotension.
C apnoea.
D transtentorial herniation.
E foraminal herniation.

282 Focal signs of intracranial lesions include:
A intellectual and emotional changes associated with parietal lobe lesions.
B astereognosis associated with parietal lobe lesions.
C bitemporal hemianopia associated with occipital lobe lesions.
D nystagmus associated with temporal lobe lesions.
E bitemporal hemianopia associated with pituitary lesions.

283 Chronic subdural haematoma:
A is usually associated with head injury.
B usually occurs in young males.
C is associated with fluctuating confusion and drowsiness.
D is more likely to occur in chronic alcoholics.
E may mimic a stroke.

284 The Glasgow Coma Scale:
A is based on four patient responses — eye opening, verbal response, motor response and pupillary reflexes.
B is 10 in a patient with a normal level of consciousness.
C defines coma as a score of 8 or less.
D if less than 8 in a trauma victim is an indication to perform exploratory burrholes.
E is used principally as a 'one-off' test to rapidly document the level of consciousness.

(Answers overleaf)

281 **A False** Bradycardia.
     B False Hypertension. Both A and B constitute 'Cushing's response'.
     C True
     D True The medial aspect of the temporal lobe is forced down through the tentorial notch, leading to compression of the aqueduct and obstruction of CSF flow.
     E True The cerebellar tonsils and medulla are displaced downwards through the foramen magnum, leading ultimately to loss of consciousness and decerebration.

282 **A False** These are associated with frontal lobe lesions.
     B True
     C False Homonymous hemianopia.
     D False With cerebellar lesions.
     E True Due to compression of the optic chiasma.

283 **A False** There is usually no history of trauma.
     B False It is a condition of the middle-aged or elderly.
     C True This is the most consistent feature.
     D True
     E True Patients with this condition are frequently to a medical ward as an atypical stroke. Hence, a CT scan should always be performed to distinguish between the two.

284 **A False** It is based on the first three of these behavioural responses.
     B False Full consciousness merits a score of 14.
     C True
     D False This simply indicates that the patient is unconscious — the cause may be an intracranial haematoma, cerebral oedema or hypotension due to a thoracic, abdominal or other injury.
     E False It is used principally as a serial test to detect changes (particularly deterioration) in the level of consciousness.

(For more information, see ch 37 of Principles and Practice of Surgery)

285 In a multiply traumatised patient who also has a head injury:

A an immediate skull X-ray is mandatory.

B immediate neurosurgical management of the head injury takes precedence over resuscitation and assessment and management of other injuries.

C a dilated and fixed pupil is inevitably associated with death of the patient.

D the pupillary response is the most important physical sign in terms of assessment of the head injury.

E intravenous dexamethasone infusion should be commenced immediately.

286 The following statements are true:

A meningocele is usually associated with a neurological deficit.

B spina bifida occulta is usually not associated with a neurological deficit.

C meningomyelocele occurs most commonly at the base of the skull.

D syringomyelia is associated with 'dissociated sensory loss'.

E spinal stenosis is a congenital generalised narrowing of the vertebral canal.

287 Subarachnoid haemorrhage:

A is usually due to atherosclerotic disease of the cerebral vessels.

B usually presents with severe headache, neck stiffness and photophobia.

C is confirmed by skull X-ray.

D should be investigated by cerebral angiography.

E may be associated with initial symptoms of vague headache or neck pain before the major presentation occurs.

(Answers overleaf)

285 A False   A skull X-ray adds exceptionally little to the initial decision-making and management. Remember, the three most important early X-rays in a multiply traumatised patient are those of the cervical spine, chest and pelvis.

B False   Despite the presence of the head injury, assessment and resuscitation follows the same (ABCDE) sequence for each patient. In a head-injured patient, early assessment and resuscitation to ensure adequate cerebral perfusion and oxygenation are as important as the definitive treatment of the intracranial lesion.

C False

D False   The level of consciousness is the most important.

E False   This may be appropriate if subsequent investigation reveals the presence of raised intracranial pressure or cerebral oedema — it is not indicated in the immediate resuscitation phase.

286 A False   There is usually no neurological deficit.

B True

C False   It occurs most commonly in the lumbar region.

D True   Loss of pain and temperature sensation, but not touch, due to involvement of the decussating pain and temperature pathways.

E True   Symptoms, related to cord compression, usually do not occur until middle age.

287 A False   It is usually due to rupture of an aneurysm (Berry aneurysm) of the cerebral vessels. It may also be due to arteriovenous malformation, trauma or tumour.

B True   This indicates meningism, as does a positive Kernig's sign.

C False   It is confirmed by lumbar puncture — the fluid is evenly blood-stained, in contrast to a 'traumatic tap', which progressively clears. Lumbar puncture has been superceded by CT scanning.

D True   To identify the exact site and cause of bleeding.

E True   So-called pre-ictal symptoms due to an initial relatively minor haemorrhage.

(For more information, see ch 37 of Principles and Practice of Surgery)

288   The following may be associated with pituitary tumours:
A   quadrantanopia.
B   multiple endocrine neoplasia (MEN) II.
C   Conn's syndrome.
D   Nelson's syndrome.
E   amenorrhoea.

289   The following statements are true:
A   approximately 50% of intracranial tumours are metastatic.
B   meningiomas frequently metastasise.
C   craniopharyngioma may result in hypopituitarism.
D   gliomas are the commonest primary brain tumours.
E   medulloblastoma usually occurs in adults.

290   The following statements are true:
A   cerebral abscess is usually due to haematogenous spread.
B   cerebral abscess often results in epilepsy.
C   Paget's disease of the skull may predispose to malignant transformation.
D   in acute head injury, a fixed dilated pupil is always caused by an intracranial haematoma.
E   chronic subdural haematoma almost never causes a visual field loss.

(Answers overleaf)

288 A True With more extensive suprasellar extension of the tumour, complete bitemporal hemianopia develops.
    B False MEN I.
    C False This refers to primary hyperaldosteronism due to a lesion in the adrenal cortex.
    D True Occurs after bilateral adrenalectomy for Cushing's disease, resulting in the development of the undetected primary pituitary adenoma. It is principally associated with hyperpigmentation.
    E True The syndrome of amenorrhoea–galactorrhoea is associated with a prolactinoma of the pituitary.

289 A True The most frequent primary sites are lung and breast.
    B False They rarely metastasise but frequently invade local vascular structures (e.g. sagittal sinus).
    C True This tumour arises in the remnant of Rathke's pouch. Progressive growth may result in hypopituitarism, due to involvement of the hypothalamus.
    D True These arise from the supporting cells of the brain (the glia) and include astrocytomas and oligodendrogliomas.
    E False This is a malignant tumour of childhood, which arises in the roof of the fourth ventricle and tends to seed via the CSF.

290 A False While this is a cause, particularly in patients with bronchiectasis or lung abscess, direct extension from the paranasal sinuses, mastoid or middle ear is the most common cause.
    B True Nearly 50% of people with cerebral abscess develop epilepsy.
    C True Osteogenic sarcoma may develop in the affected bone.
    D False It may be caused by cerebral oedema.
    E True

(For more information, see ch 37 of Principles and Practice of Surgery)

30. Practical procedures

291 Concerning surgical scrub and skin preparation:
- **A** the principal aim is to kill all the resident skin flora.
- **B** hand washing with soap and water alone results in an increased viable bacterial count on the skin.
- **C** alcohol is a more potent and rapid skin disinfectant than both iodine and chlorhexidine.
- **D** alcohol has a potent residual activity on skin flora.
- **E** iodine is most active at normal body pH.

292 In wound closure:
- **A** atraumatic round-bodied needles are used in skin closure.
- **B** where local anaesthesia is employed, 30 ml of 1% lignocaine is a safe dose in a 70 kg adult.
- **C** local anaesthetic with 1 in 200 000 adrenaline affords longer anaesthetic time, making it useful for ring blocks in the fingers and toes.
- **D** non-absorbable suture material is necessary for closing the anterior sheath in the abdominal wall, if wound dehiscence and incisional hernia are to be avoided.
- **E** sutures on the face and neck should be removed early for the best cosmetic result.

(Answers overleaf)

291 A False This is impossible. Human skin flora can be divided into two types: resident flora, which colonise the skin almost continuously; and transient flora, which are present for only short periods. Therefore the aim of the preoperative surgical scrub is to kill the transient flora and reduce the resident flora in order to reduce the risk of wound contamination.

B True The resident flora exist on the skin in microcolonies, often extending deep into sweat glands, sebaceous glands and hair follicles, hence normal hand washing may only serve to expose the resident flora and increase surface bacterial counts.

C True Alcohols reduce viable bacterial counts by 95%, compared with 70–80% for chlorhexidine and povidone-iodine. The alcohols are the most rapidly bactericidal and are effective in the rapid disinfection of transient flora.

D False Alcohol acts by denaturing protein. Its only weak points are the safety aspects and it has no residual activity.

E False Iodine is most active at an acid pH (<4).

292 A False Cutting needles are necessary to penetrate the tough dermis. Round-bodied needles are ideal for subcutaneous closure and for intestinal anastomoses.

B False The recommended safe dose is <3 mg/kg. In the example given, the safe dose would be <210 mg. A 1% solution of lignocaine contains 10 mg/ml, hence the patient would be receiving a dose of 300 mg.

C False It is hazardous to use it in sites where there are end arteries, such as the digits, nose, ear lobes and penis.

D False Wound dehiscence and incisional hernia occurrence is not related to suture strength but to other variables, such as surgical technique and patient problems (persistently raised intra-abdominal pressure, impaired healing, anaemia, jaundice, malnourishment, scurvy, diabetes and Cushing's syndrome).

E True The face and neck have an excellent blood supply and heal quickly.

(For more information, see ch 38 of Principles and Practice of Surgery)

293 A nasogastric tube:
A employed for drainage of gastric contents in the immediate postoperative period is most effective if it has a double lumen.
B which is 16 FG (French gauge) has an internal diameter of 1.6 mm.
C is essential in the head-injured patient to prevent aspiration pnemonitis.
D used for enteral feeding should be aspirated to confirm the site of placement prior to the commencement of feeding.
E when being inserted usually meets most resistance around 10 cm from the anterior nares.

294 The Sengstaken–Blakemore tube:
A is used in the emergency management of bleeding oesophageal varices.
B is a double-lumen tube.
C is currently the most commonly employed strategy in the management of bleeding oesophageal varices.
D has an oesophageal balloon which should be inflated to 70 mmHg to overcome the portal hypertension in the tributaries of the coronary and left gastric veins.
E should always be inserted by the oral route.

295 Retrieval of intraperitoneal fluid:
A is of value in assessing the need for laparotomy following closed abdominal trauma.
B has a high sensitivity and specificity in the diagnosis of malignant ascites.
C which has a protein content of <30 g/l could be due to cardiac or hepatic failure.
D is of value in determining the severity of acute pancreatitis.
E may improve the mental state of patients with hepatic encephalopathy.

(Answers overleaf)

293 A True   This is the principle of a sump tube.
    B False   French gauge refers not to the internal diameter of the tube but to the circumference in millimetres.
    C False   Nasogastric tubes are potentially dangerous in head-injured patients: (a) at insertion if facial fractures are present, and (b) as they may introduce sepsis into the central nervous system.
    D False   Nasogastric tubes used in enteral feeding are usually very fine and collapse on aspiration. Position is checked by X-ray.
    E False   The point of most resistance is the cricopharyngeus muscle at 20 cm from the incisors/anterior nares.

294 A True
    B False   It has four — one to inflate the gastric balloon, one to inflate the oesophageal balloon, one to aspirate the pharynx and oesophagus, and one to aspirate the stomach or administer drugs.
    C False   Its main role is in the stabilisation of patients prior to injection of varices or for transfer to a regional unit. Sandostatin (octreotide) infusion is the mainstay of treatment and acts by reducing splanchnic blood flow and portal pressure.
    D False   The oesophageal balloon need only be inflated to 40 mmHg to achieve adequate variceal tamponade.
    E False   It is not contraindicated to insert the tube by the oral route, but it is usually inserted via the nasopharynx.

295 A True   A red blood cell count of >100 000/ml, white cell count of >500/ml, and amylase count of >175u/ml are suggestive of significant intra-abdominal injury and a laparotomy should be performed. This test has a diagnostic accuracy of >90%.
    B False   In only 50% of cases where there is malignant ascites will a diagnostic tap for cytological confirmation be successful.
    C True   This is the diagnostic criterion for a transudate. Hepatic or cardiac failure are common causes of transudate formation.
    D True   A prune-coloured aspirate is of bad prognostic significance.
    E False   A large volume of fluid (>2 litres) aspirated from a patient with hepatic failure may precipitate hepatic encephalopathy.

(For more information, see ch 38 of Principles and Practice of Surgery)

296 Tracheostomy:

A may be performed percutaneously using the Seldinger technique.

B is most commonly indicated in patients requiring prolonged ventilatory support.

C in the emergency situation has been superseded by cricothyroidotomy.

D should avoid the first tracheal ring as this predisposes to subglottic stenosis.

E which is temporary will require formal surgical closure.

297 Chest drain insertion:

A does not require observation of a full aseptic technique.

B is unnecessary in spontaneous pneumothoraces of less than 50%.

C is associated with fewer complications when performed under direct vision with blunt dissection down to the parietal pleura.

D is not indicated in malignant pleural effusions.

E should be in the intercostal space at the lower border of the rib.

(Answers overleaf)

296 A True   This is being performed increasingly by anaesthetists and has been shown to be a very efficacious method with few complications.

B True   The main indications for tracheostomy are: (1) to prevent tracheal stenosis in patients requiring prolonged ventilation; (2) to bypass an obstruction in the upper airway; (3) to provide continuous access to the lower airway.

C True   A needle may be introduced through the crico-thyroid membrane between the thyroid cartilage and first tracheal ring, and the airway maintained until a formal tracheostomy is performed.

D True   Damage to the first tracheal ring predisposes not only to subglottic stenosis but also to tracheo-innominate artery fistula.

E. False   A dry dressing is sufficient as tracheostomy wounds close well by secondary intention.

297 A False   A full aseptic technique should be observed, local anaesthetic infiltrated and, depending on the specific situation, the site should be carefully considered.

B False   If the pneumothorax is less than 30% then an expectant policy can be adopted, but it is important to re-X-ray the chest after 12 hours to ensure that the pneumothorax is not enlarging.

C True   This is the method recommended in most thoracic units; it is associated with less bleeding, negates misplacement of the drain and lowers the risk of pulmonary contusion.

D False   The pleural cavity can be drained more completely prior to performing pleurodesis using sclerosants.

E False   The intercostal neurovascular bundle lies at the lower border, and bleeding is likely if the drain is introduced in this site. It is more appropriate to insert the drain as close to the upper border of the rib as possible.

(For more information, see ch 38 of Principles and Practice of Surgery)

298 Chest drains:
   A should follow the most direct route from skin to pleural cavity if complications are to be avoided.
   B should be at least 32 FG and placed basally for the effective treatment of large pneumothoraces.
   C which persistently bubble profusely suggest a bronchopleural fistula.
   D for treatment of uncomplicated pneumothoraces seldom require to be left in situ for more than 24 hours.
   E should be inserted with prophylactic antibiotic cover.

299 Central venous catheterisation:
   A may be used to estimate the intravascular volume.
   B is commonly employed for administration of parenteral nutrition.
   C via the right internal jugular vein is associated with thoracic duct injury.
   D using a subcutaneous tunnel lowers the incidence of line sepsis.
   E should only be performed with ECG monitoring.

300 Lumbar puncture:
   A is useful in the diagnosis of subarachnoid haemorrhage.
   B involves the insertion of a fine needle into the subdural space.
   C should be performed with the patient in the prone position.
   D may have fatal consequences if performed in communicating hydrocephalus.
   E is part of the septic work-up in an infant with unexplained pyrexia.

(Answers overleaf)

298 A False   An oblique tract aids primary union of the wound, reduces the risk of infection and decreases air entry into the pleural space when the tube is removed.

B False   For pneumothoraces it is sufficient to use a small-gauge drain (28 FG), which should be directed apically. 32 FG drains placed basally are employed to drain thick pus or clotted blood.

C True   This is the classical presentation. The initial treatment is to apply low-grade suction to the chest drain; this encourages not only re-expansion of the lung but also closure of the fistula.

D True   Most pneumothoraces will respond to 24 hours of chest drainage, at which time the tube should be removed as the patient expires fully and an occlusive dressing should be applied.

E False   Although the risk of empyema is 3% there is no indication for the use of prophylactic antibiotics.

299 A True   The central venous catheter may be used to measure the central venous pressure which, in the absence of heart failure, will give an estimation of the circulating blood volume.

B True   It is necessary to deliver such hyperosmolar solutions into a large central vein where the dilutional effect will reduce the risk of thrombophlebitis and thrombosis.

C False   The right internal jugular approach does not endanger the thoracic duct, which is situated on the left side.

D True

E True   If passed into the right ventricle, it can initiate ventricular fibrillation.

300 A True   In the era before CT scanning, lumbar puncture and the presence of xanthochromia was diagnostic.

B False   This is the epidural space. The arachnoid mater requires to be penetrated before the subarachnoid space is entered.

C False   This is very rare. The patient is normally positioned in the left lateral position with the spine flexed and the needle is inserted between the L3/L4 interspace.

D False   Raised intracranial pressure is not an absolute contraindication to lumbar puncture but is very dangerous when non-communicating hydrocephalus exists.

E True   Septic work-up involves blood culture, urine culture and lumbar puncture with examination of the CSF.

(For more information, see ch 38 of Principles and Practice of Surgery)

Principles and Practice of Surgery

The surgery textbook you can trust

New Edition!

Edited by

A P M Forrest, D C Carter, I B Macleod

1995   Third edition   642 pages   300 line and 100 halftone illus
ISBN 0 443 04860 6

Principles and Practice of Surgery, 3rd edition, is a comprehensive, disease-based textbook of surgery, ordered by body systems, which has been fully updated in both content and approach to avoid overburdening you with large amounts of non-essential information. The text enables you to appreciate both the medical and surgical implications of diseases encountered in surgical wards.

Written and edited by a team of highly-experienced teaching and operating surgeons, with students' needs in mind, the book also contains additional contributions from experts on specialist aspects of surgery.

How new design features convey information memorably...

- The page layout has been redesigned and a second colour added for greater clarity
- Summary boxes are now included to aid revision
- Radiographs have been introduced to reflect the increasing emphasis on surgical diagnosis by investigation
- The line illustrations have been revised to convey information more clearly
- Radiographs and clinical photographs have been added to show conditions realistically

References to the textbook in **MCQ Tutorial for Principles and Practice of Surgery** make it easy to follow up specific topics for more detail. Together the books are ideal for learning and revision.

Churchill Livingstone books are available from all academic bookshops, but in case of difficulty please contact:

UK only
FREEPHONE 0500 556 242
FREEPOST, Churchill Livingstone, Robert Stevenson House,
1–3 Baxter's Place, Leith Walk, EDINBURGH EH1 0BA
Elsewhere
Phone +44 (0) 131 535 1021
Fax +44 (0) 131 535 1022
Churchill Livingstone, Robert Stevenson House,
1–3 Baxter's Place, Leith Walk, EDINBURGH EH1 3AF, UK

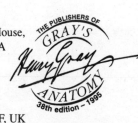
THE PUBLISHERS OF GRAY'S ANATOMY · 38th edition – 1995